Strengths of Dyscalculia

Learning from the Lived Experiences of Twice Exceptional Adults

Ashleigh D'Aunoy

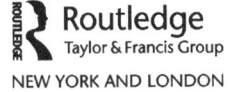
Routledge
Taylor & Francis Group
NEW YORK AND LONDON

Designed cover image: © Getty Images

First published 2026
by Routledge
605 Third Avenue, New York, NY 10158

and by Routledge
4 Park Square, Milton Park, Abingdon, Oxon, OX14 4RN

Routledge is an imprint of the Taylor & Francis Group, an informa business

© 2026 Ashleigh D'Aunoy

The right of Ashleigh D'Aunoy to be identified as author of this work has been asserted in accordance with sections 77 and 78 of the Copyright, Designs and Patents Act 1988.

All rights reserved. No part of this book may be reprinted or reproduced or utilised in any form or by any electronic, mechanical, or other means, now known or hereafter invented, including photocopying and recording, or in any information storage or retrieval system, without permission in writing from the publishers.

Trademark notice: Product or corporate names may be trademarks or registered trademarks, and are used only for identification and explanation without intent to infringe.

ISBN: 978-1-032-86502-7 (hbk)
ISBN: 978-1-032-86496-9 (pbk)
ISBN: 978-1-003-52780-0 (ebk)

DOI: 10.4324/9781003527800

Typeset in Palatino
by Apex CoVantage, LLC

Contents

Foreword..*vii*
Preface ....*ix*
Acknowledgements......................................*xi*

1 Introduction..1

2 What Do We Know?.....................................11

3 Profiles 28

4 Themes and Stories 49

5 Lessons Learned 97

6 Tips, Strategies, and Suggestions 115

7 Conclusion..136

About the Author *143*

Strengths of Dyscalculia

Strengths of Dyscalculia opens the door to reframing dyscalculia not as a deficit, but as a cognitive difference with unique strengths, offering a fresh, strength-based perspective rooted in positive psychology.

Packed with practical insights, this book provides actionable strategies to foster psychological safety, reduce math anxiety, and nurture strengths alongside addressing challenges. Through a qualitative study of gifted adults with dyscalculia, the book delves into their lived experiences, exploring the challenges they faced in educational systems ill-equipped to support their dual exceptionality, the impact on their self-concept, and the strategies they developed to navigate daily life.

Whether you're an educator, parent, researcher, or someone navigating dyscalculia yourself, this book advocates for a transformative shift in understanding and addressing dyscalculia—celebrating neurodiversity, fostering inclusive environments, and empowering twice-exceptional individuals to thrive inside the classroom and out.

Ashleigh D'Aunoy is Director of Enrichment, Innovation, and Talent Development at the Episcopal School of Acadiana where she works to meet the needs of the school's diverse learners through a strength-based, talent-focused lens. This book is based on firsthand research conducted for her dissertation.

Foreword

The author and I enjoy a mutual appreciation for sake, and we both appreciate and enjoy the beauty of mathematics—over the years we've had many wonderful conversations about math. I met Ashleigh D'Aunoy when she came to her first of many of my teacher training sessions. She was the kind of educator who was willing to put aside procedural knowledge and really embrace conceptual knowledge in teaching—in other words, the *know why* instead of the *know how*. That kind of thinking is at the heart of good math teaching, and it shows up throughout this book.

I was fortunate enough to be invited to serve on Ashleigh's dissertation committee. There's been a lot of important work on learning differences like dyslexia and dysgraphia, but not enough on dyscalculia. Her dissertation stood out—for the content and how it was written. Usually, most people hate reading a dissertation unless it's their own, but hers was absolutely beautiful and I enjoyed reading it—I never put it down once. Reading her dissertation was like reading a story, and I learned a lot. I had been tutoring a student with dyscalculia at the time, and it gave me a new perspective.

I'm tutoring a boy now who struggles even with the basics. If I say to him, "What's 4 + 3?" it takes him a long time to figure it out—even with his fingers. But his spatial skills are absolutely wonderful. Many of the students that I've worked with who seem to have dyscalculia are like that—they can't do math, but they are very good at other things. So that's where I start. I jump to the stuff they *can* do, and it's usually artistic or something they can do with their hands, like mathematical art or mathematical origami, or whatever works for them.

I've taught mathematics for over six decades now, half of that in teacher training programs, and I can confidently say: this book should be required reading in every math methods class.

You can't "fix" dyscalculia, but you can give kids the tools and support they need to work with it.

Ashleigh offers a new, necessary way to understand dyscalculia. She shows a different perspective, one that comes from deep understanding, real experience, and with ideas you can actually use. Her work reminds us: the goal isn't to fix what's *wrong*, it's to recognize what's *right* and build from there. This book does exactly that.

—Rachel McAnallen, PhD

Preface

The seed of the idea fell into my lap quite unexpectedly. I'd recently been pulled out of a third-grade classroom in a small independent school to design and implement what would eventually become our design thinking program. I was feeling unmoored without a homeroom to call my own and struggling to find ways to connect with colleagues and students while spending the bulk of my time researching design thinking, planning the physical space, and ordering supplies and materials.

My school has a pull-out learning center program that provides support for high-ability students with significant challenges due to learning disabilities. This was the first year that the learning center offered a pull-out class for math, but the teacher hired for this position unexpectedly left early in the year to join her husband who had been transferred out of state. Scrambling to find someone to take over for the two students being served, the head of the school approached me and asked if I would be willing to take over until someone else could be hired. I'd earned a reputation as a third-grade teacher for success with struggling math students and for creating a less stressful environment for those with math anxiety, both of which I attribute to my own lifelong struggles with math.

A temporary fill-in became a couple of years of working with these students, both of whom were identified as being gifted with dyscalculia. During the time I worked with them, I was continually baffled by their unique struggles. They showed growth, yes, but the roadblocks were significant and fascinating. Why was this boy unable to figure out $3 + 1$, but he could solve two-digit subtraction in a heartbeat? Why could this girl solve complex math logic problems but couldn't multiply? In my efforts to figure out a way to teach them, I was frequently frustrated by the lack of useful information available.

Around the same time, I began working toward a doctor of education in cognitive diversity through Bridges Graduate School of Cognitive Diversity in Education, a first-of-its kind graduate program focusing on twice-exceptional education through a strength-based, talent-focused lens. I remember taking one of the first courses of my doctoral program, "Introduction to Cognitively Diverse Minds," with Dr. Susan Baum. I looked forward to learning more about the strengths of differently wired brains and especially about dyscalculia. To my surprise and dismay, dyscalculia was not part of the course, and it wasn't represented in any of the many articles and books we were assigned.

My dissertation research grew from that frustration. I was determined to shine a light on dyscalculia and bring it into those conversations we were having about the benefits and strengths of neurodiversity. This book is based on that dissertation.

Acknowledgements

First and foremost, I'd like to thank those individuals—Susan Baum, Rachel McAnallen, C. Matthew Fugate, Thomas Hébert, Enyi Jen, and Jade Rivera—who believed that my dissertation was worthy of a wider audience, encouraged me to write a book, and supported me through the process.

Because this book began as a dissertation, this acknowledgement would be incomplete without mentioning my advisor and committee members: Karen Westberg, whose honest and specific feedback guided and elevated the quality of my work; Robin Schader, whose expertise, command of the rules of writing, and keen and critical eye helped immensely, especially in the final stages of editing; and Rachel McAnallen, whose insight, depth of understanding of the nuances of math learning, positive energy, and humor first inspired me—a math-anxious and math-averse student turned educator—to transform my teaching practice to become a more skilled and effective math teacher, especially for those who struggle.

I am so thankful for the insights of my capable editor, Rebecca Collazo, and editorial assistant, Quinn Cowen. I was completely in the dark on how all of this book stuff works, and your positivity, encouragement, and guidance carried me through.

Writing a book sometimes felt like a monumental task, so I am forever grateful for the friends and family who sustained me through this process by offering words of encouragement, celebrating benchmarks, serving as sounding boards, helping me stay accountable, and just letting me be me: Jade Rivera, Holly Kincaid, Michelle Haj-Broussard, and Lara Greene. Extra thanks to Christine Adams, Leslie Boudreaux-Tidwell, and Kathleen O'Shaughnessy for being the best and most enthusiastic cheerleaders I could have asked for. Our group texts always have and will continue to be bright spots in my days.

All of this work stems from my experiences with all of my students, present and past, and I owe a big thanks to all of them for challenging me to be a better teacher and to want to understand more. An especially big thank you to the students referenced in Chapter 1: your brilliance and your struggles and my frustration with a lack of strength-based descriptions of and resources for dyscalculia to better serve you led me down this path.

This book would not have been possible without the contributions of my research participants: James, Emma, Amelia, Sylvia, and Louisa. Thank you all for trusting me with your stories.

Thank you to my parents, Ronald and Marsha D'Aunoy, for instilling in me a love of learning and a need to follow my curiosity. If she was still with us, my mother would have been so proud to brag about her published daughter to all of her friends.

And lastly, much love to my husband, Paul Conover, and to my son, Julien Conover. Thank you both for your love and support and for giving me space to try to be my best self.

1

Introduction

Picture a boy, ten years old, highly gifted in language, with extensive knowledge of history and talent in music but who cannot accurately count the 20 small cubes in front of him because he has not yet developed one-to-one correspondence. Now imagine a seven-year-old girl, bright, with a sharp wit and above-average logical reasoning, who struggles to skip count, even by fives and tens, because she cannot recognize and apply patterns in numbers. These two students are diagnosed with dyscalculia, and these skills and concepts, as well as others that can be troublesome for them, such as subitization, number sense, place value, and more, are the foundation upon which more complex math understanding rests. Essential foundational math skills are usually acquired during early childhood, but without a solid bedrock, students with dyscalculia fall further and further behind.

Dyscalculia is a learning difference that is largely unknown and poorly understood (Butterworth, 2019). In addition, and unlike other more commonly known learning differences such as dyslexia, attention deficit hyperactivity disorder (ADHD), and autism spectrum disorder (ASD), where an understanding of the strengths of these kinds of brains is beginning to be recognized, a substantial body of knowledge around the brain wiring of dyscalculia does not seem to exist. Without this knowledge, questions about the potential strengths of dyscalculia (for example, in the way that students with ADHD often display higher divergent thinking ability) are as yet unanswered. As a result, rather than

DOI: 10.4324/9781003527800-1

being rooted in scientific understanding and with a focus on strengths, math instruction for students with dyscalculia is deficit based and tends to focus on rote learning, repetition, and other "tried-and-true" methods. Many issues further cloud and compound this lack of recognition and understanding: co-occurring conditions; widespread math anxiety among students, parents, and teachers; teacher attitudes toward learning differences; and the problems associated with an ineffective adoption of the Common Core Standards, to name a few. Furthermore, and contrary to attitudes about reading and writing, it is socially acceptable for someone to identify as "bad at math" or "not a math person." As a result, there is often less motivation on the part of parents to seek support for their children, except in very extreme circumstances, such as looming failure of a course or grade level. If teachers are to support and grow students with dyscalculia, research is needed to inform effective strategies.

Some may argue that existing methods of instruction are sufficient to address these learners' needs. Strategies such as the concrete-representational-abstract (CRA) model and use of manipulatives are examples of best practices with clear benefits for many students (Boggan et al., 2010; Witzel et al., 2008). Additionally, progress has been made in addressing effective ways to teach students with math anxiety (Blazer, 2011). Others assert that repetition and skills practice are essential for students who struggle in math. Many teachers swear by these methods, and many students have shown remarkable progress with these approaches. However, in the face of fundamental breakdowns in a student's ability to move through the developmental phases of math skills and concepts acquisition, these strategies, though indeed rooted in best practices and shown to be successful, yield inconsistent results for students with dyscalculia.

Twice-Exceptional/2e and a Strength-Based Lens

Twice exceptional, or 2e, individuals are those with potential for high achievement or creative productivity in one or more domains who also have one or more learning disabilities (Reis et al., 2014).

Twice exceptional can also be referred to as gifted with learning disabilities (Baum et al., 2017). Lack of understanding about giftedness contributes to a lack of understanding about 2e. Aren't gifted people smart? Why would they struggle?

Twice-exceptionality is a complex and often misunderstood topic—whole books have been written about the subject. For our purposes here, important points to be aware of are:

- Giftedness and learning differences/disabilities can coexist.
  - A gifted individual can also be diagnosed with dyscalculia, ADHD, dyslexia, autism, dysgraphia, and others, as well as any combination.
- Identification can be challenging.
  - Strengths can mask challenges, challenges can mask strengths, or strengths and challenges can mask each other.
- Dual exceptionalities require dual support.
  - In order to thrive academically, socially, and emotionally, 2e individuals require opportunities to develop their strengths and talents, as well as support for their struggles.

Strength-based, talent-focused learning is a teaching practice that focuses on strengths and talents of 2e students and de-emphasizes their disabilities, which allows students' gifted characteristics to become more apparent and which leads to increased engagement and success (Reis et al., 2014). Research in strength-based learning has demonstrated benefits for all students and is essential for those who are 2e. These benefits include increased motivation and engagement; a more positive sense of self; and academic, social, and emotional growth (Baum et al., 2017).

In spite of the compelling evidence in support of a strength-based approach, teaching for students with dyscalculia is largely deficit based, which negatively affects a student's confidence and ability to engage in and make progress in math class. Better understanding of dyscalculia and a shift away from a deficit lens could provide a solid, research-backed foundation for effective teaching strategies.

Lack of data and research supports the need for further investigation into dyscalculia. A knowledge base about the ways that math is processed for students with dyscalculia, set within a framework of understanding the developmental stages for the acquisition of math skills and concepts, coupled with identification of potential strengths of those with this learning difference and viewed through a strength-based learning lens, would provide a solid foundation on which to create more reliable teaching strategies for this population. More importantly, a strength-based perspective of dyscalculia could have far-reaching implications for development of a more positive self-concept for these students.

What Is Dyscalculia?

Dyscalculia is a learning difference related to a person's ability to subitize, estimate, and compare quantities, and these challenges can be further complicated by other factors that negatively affect success, such as math anxiety, among others (Knop & Chou, 2020). According to Butterworth (2019), dyscalculia affects approximately 4–7% of students; however, my own experience and conversations with colleagues in education and educational psychology suggest that many teachers are unaware of dyscalculia and therefore unable to recognize it or provide appropriate support for those students. Research and understanding of dyscalculia have not kept pace with the advances in understanding of other learning differences, such as dyslexia, ADHD, and ASD. For many of these learning differences, there is a growing understanding of the benefits of those diverse brain wirings; however, there is limited knowledge about the brain wiring and potential positive characteristics of dyscalculia. As a result, dyscalculia is viewed through the medical model as a problem to be fixed, and teaching strategies are not rooted in scientific research or a strength-based approach.

Goals

This research is important for its contribution to advancing understanding of dyscalculia and laying a foundation for this learning difference to be accepted as a cognitive difference with its own set of strengths, rather than as a deficit to be fixed. A reframing of dyscalculia through the lens of its strengths paves the way for further study, including neuroimaging studies, to reinforce and provide evidence for strengths and the development of effective teaching strategies that are based in scientific research. Most significantly, the research will allow those with dyscalculia to develop a more positive self-concept, which will support increased engagement and motivation and lead to successes rather than failures.

In addition to advancing understanding, this research aims to support meaningful, real-world change by offering practical strategies rooted in a strength-based perspective. By including concrete suggestions for students, parents, and educators, the book connects research to practice, providing tools that can be applied in school, work, and everyday life. These suggested strategies are intended not only to foster success but also to call attention to the capabilities and potential of dyscalculic individuals.

Research Study Nuts and Bolts

This book grew from a dissertation titled *Strengths of Dyscalculia: A Multiple Case Study Analysis of Gifted Adults*, completed for the degree of doctor of education in cognitive diversity in 2023. Unlike quantitative research, which analyzes numerical data, this study was qualitative, which focuses on descriptive data, such as from interviews and/or observations, to draw conclusions about perceptions, experiences, and meaning. This particular study followed a case study approach, which "investigates a contemporary phenomenon within its real-life context" (Yin, 2014, as cited in Merriam & Tisdell, 2016). Through this approach, it is possible to analyze data within and across different contexts, which supports synthesis of similarities, differences, and patterns between multiple cases (Baxter & Jack, 2008; Stake, 2006).

In this study, the phenomena studied were the academic, cognitive, socioemotional, and creative strengths of gifted adults with dyscalculia. The goal was to examine the experiences and perceptions of the participants and to determine how their identity as both gifted and dyscalculic has shaped those experiences and perceptions as well as allowed them to find their niche in life.

A qualitative research study is guided by research questions, which for this study included:

1. What are the academic, cognitive, social, emotional, and creative strengths of adults who have been identified as gifted and diagnosed with dyscalculia?
2. What academic, social, and extracurricular experiences of gifted adults with dyscalculia supported development of their strengths?
3. What academic, social, emotional, and extracurricular experiences of gifted adults with dyscalculia affected their ability to overcome academic, social, emotional, and cognitive challenges?
4. How do gifted adults with dyscalculia navigate math-related challenges in their personal and professional lives?

To control the scope of the study, potential participants were required to meet specific selection criteria, which included the following: (1) all participants were 18 years old or older; (2) all participants had evidence of high ability in one or more domains, such as through testing and formal identification of giftedness or other tangible evidence; (3) all participants had a documented diagnosis of dyscalculia or an equivalent diagnosis, such as specific learning disorder with impairment in math; and (4) all participants agreed to participate in interviews and any follow-up interviews.

Estimates of the percentage of individuals who are 2e are small, as are estimates of the percentage of individuals with dyscalculia. As a result, finding participants who met the criteria for a study about a little-known learning difference among a small 2e population proved to be a challenge. Participants were recruited in a variety of ways. Some were solicited from professors, colleagues, and educational psychologists specializing in dyscalculia among 2e individuals. Other participants were recruited from among members of social media groups dedicated to dyscalculia and the 2e community. After receiving fewer than a dozen responses, six individuals were identified as meeting the criteria and interviewed, and five of those were then selected for further analysis. One participant was excluded from the study due to uncertainty about meeting the selection criteria, and the participant did not respond to follow-up questions seeking clarification. This participant was also excluded due to a lack of data about experiences with math in school.

Interviews, which were conducted through video conferencing, lasted one to two hours and took place between August 2022 and January 2023. Each interview followed a semistructured format with most questions planned in advance. A semistructured format ensures that specific topics are addressed, provides a framework for organization and clarity, and allows for flexibility as needed (Merriam & Tisdell, 2016). Over the course of the interviews, some questions were modified and new questions emerged, including questions regarding the role of creativity as a strength. Follow-up questions after the initial interview were conducted through email and included questions intended to solicit additional details about specific responses, as well as additional demographic information.

Transcriptions were created in real time during interviews with the support of artificial intelligence (AI) and were edited immediately following each interview for accuracy. Each participant also received copies of their transcript to check for accuracy and to offer any clarification or additional thoughts. Confidentiality is important in a research study. Each participant's identity is protected through the use of pseudonyms and removal of identifying information.

Data analysis consisted of multiple levels of coding and cross-case analysis, which allowed for identification of similarities and

TABLE 1.1 Common themes identified in participant interviews

Themes
Strengths of adults with dyscalculia
Opportunities to develop strengths and interests
Support received during schooling
Emotional and behavioral responses
Math struggles
Strategies for navigating adult challenges

differences among the cases. Six common themes were identified (see Table 1.1). Finally, naturalistic generalizations were developed to determine what generalizations could be applied to the population being studied (Creswell & Poth, 2018).

What's in the Book?

This first chapter serves as an introduction by presenting a rationale for the research, laying a foundation for understanding of 2e and a strength-based approach to provide context for the study, outlining how the study was conducted, and presenting an overview of what the book hopes to accomplish. Chapter 2 sums up important ideas and information from existing research (what would be the review of the literature in a dissertation) relevant to dyscalculia, twice-exceptionality, and a strength-based, talent-focused approach. This chapter will also briefly address language and terminology choices and related issues of accessibility. Chapter 3 offers a brief overview of the participants in the study to provide context. Chapters 4 and 5 are the heart of the book—the stories and lessons learned of the adults who participated in the research study, all of whom have gifts and talents in a variety of areas and have experienced, and continue to experience, significant challenges as a result of dyscalculia. Research and data are important, but parents, teachers, and individuals want concrete strategies. With this mind, Chapter 6 presents tips and strategies drawn from the participants, personal experience, and other sources, as well as support for advocacy in school, the workplace, and life. Finally, the conclusion in Chapter 7 sums it all up and gives suggestions for where to go from here.

Conclusion

By closely investigating the lived experiences of gifted adults with dyscalculia, this book hopes to reframe attitudes about dyscalculia from a deficit-based to a strength-based lens and lay a foundation for further strength-based research into this little-known and commonly misunderstood learning difference. If you, the reader, are looking for fresh perspectives on dyscalculia, this book is for you. If you have struggled with dyscalculia yourself, or care about someone who has, or if you work with 2e students or dyscalculic students in particular, this book has something for you.

This book offers the opportunity for increased empathy and deeper understanding, as well as practical tools and strategies to foster confidence and increase potential through real stories, evidence-based insights, and actionable strategies. Discover how recognizing the strengths of dyscalculia can transform how we understand, value, teach, and empower individuals who experience math in all its forms in unique and challenging ways.

References

Baum, S. M., Schader, R., & Owen, S. (2017). *To be gifted and learning disabled: Strength-based strategies for helping twice-exceptional students with LD, ADHD, and more.* Prufrock Press. https://www.routledge.com/To-Be-Gifted-and-Learning-Disabled-Strength-Based-Strategies-for-Helping/Baum-Schader-Owen/p/book/9781618216441

Baxter, P., & Jack, S. (2008). Qualitative case study methodology: Study design and implementation for novice researchers. *The Qualitative Report, 13*(4), 544–559. https://nsuworks.nova.edu/tqr/vol13/iss4/2

Blazer, C. (2011). *Strategies for reducing math anxiety* (Vol. 1102). Research Services Information Capsule, Miami-Dade County Public School. https://eric.ed.gov/?id=ED536509

Boggan, M., Harper, S., & Whitmire, A. (2010). Using manipulatives to teach elementary mathematics. *Journal of Instructional Pedagogies, 3*, 1–6. https://eric.ed.gov/?id=EJ1096945

Butterworth, B. (2019). *Dyscalculia: From science to education.* Routledge. https://www.routledge.com/Dyscalculia-from-Science-to-Education/Butterworth/p/book/9781138688612

Creswell, J. W., & Poth, C. N. (2018). *Qualitative inquiry and research design: Choosing among five approaches.* Sage. https://us.sagepub.com/en-us/nam/qualitative-inquiry-and-research-design/book246896

D'Aunoy, A. (2023). *Strengths of dyscalculia: A multiple case study analysis of gifted adults* (Order No. 30692919). Available from ProQuest Central; ProQuest Dissertations & Theses Global. (2892615561). https://www.proquest.com/dissertations-theses/strengths-dyscalculia-multiple-case-study/docview/2892615561/se-2

Knop, N. F., & Chou, S. H. (2020). Giftedness and math difficulty. In C. M. Fugate, W. Behrens, & C. Boswell (Eds.), *Understanding twice exceptional learners: Connecting research to practice* (pp. 183–216). Prufrock Press. https://www.routledge.com/Understanding-Twice-Exceptional-Learners-Connecting-Research-to-Practice/Fugate-Behrens-Boswell/p/book/9781646320776

Merriam, S. B., & Tisdell, E. J. (2016). *Qualitative research: A guide to design and implementation.* Jossey-Bass. https://www.wiley.com/en-us/Qualitative+Research:+A+Guide+to+Design+and+Implementation,+4th+Edition-p-9781119003618

Reis, S. M., Baum, S. M., & Burke, E. (2014). An operational definition of twice-exceptional learners: Implications and applications. *Gifted Child Quarterly, 58*, 217–230. https://journals.sagepub.com/doi/abs/10.1177/0016986214534976

Stake, R. E. (2006). *Multiple case study analysis.* The Guilford Press. https://www.routledge.com/Multiple-Case-Study-Analysis/Stake/p/book/9781593852481

Witzel, B. S., Riccomini, P. J., & Schneider, E. (2008). Implementing CRA with secondary students with learning disabilities in mathematics. *Intervention in School and Clinic, 43*(5), 270–276. https://journals.sagepub.com/doi/10.1177/1053451208314734

2
What Do We Know?

An important step in a research study is to take a deep dive into the existing research to uncover what is already known or understood, identify gaps, and provide context for the study. Here, that information is presented to provide a framework for understanding the study itself. The summary of the research on dyscalculia and other topics relevant to the study is organized into six sections: (1) definitions and diagnostic criteria; (2) subtypes of dyscalculia; (3) complexities and co-occurring conditions; (4) neuroscientific research; (5) twice-exceptionality; and (6) a strength-based, talent-focused lens of dyscalculia. This review also presents the theoretical framework used in the study and shines a spotlight on the gaps in research and understanding, particularly about the strengths associated with this learning difference.

A note about learning *differences* versus learning *disabilities*. There are debate and differing preferences on the choice of these overlapping, but different terms. *Learning differences* places emphasis on natural human variation, but with this choice, there is a risk of minimizing the very real, often disabling challenges that individuals face. In my professional life, I try to consider context when choosing which terminology to use. In a dissertation or a book, however, consistency is important. I chose to use learning difference, rather than disability, because the focus of the study was on identifying strengths and reframing dyscalculia as a cognitive difference.

DOI: 10.4324/9781003527800-2

Definitions and Diagnostic Criteria

As understanding of other learning differences has grown, an understanding of learning differences related to math are lagging far behind (Butterworth, 2019; Gersten et al., 2005). There is little consensus among researchers on definitions or cognitive factors of dyscalculia and on diagnostic criteria (Mazzocco & Myers, 2003; Szucs & Goswani, 2013). Additionally, different terminology is used throughout the literature, which includes dyscalculia or developmental dyscalculia (Butterworth, 2019; Kosc, 1974), specific learning disorder with impairment in mathematics (American Psychiatric Association, 2017), and mathematical learning disability or MD (Geary, 2004; Mazzocco & Myers, 2003). Adding to the confusion of terminology is the diagnostic criteria for identification, which can vary widely (Butterworth, 2019). Furthermore, mathematical development and acquisition of skills are complex, which clouds attempts to make sense of associated learning differences (Geary, 2004).

Butterworth's definition is based on Kosc's (1974) who first used the term developmental dyscalculia, which he defined as a

> [S]tructural disorder of mathematical abilities which has its origin in a genetic or congenital disorder of those parts of the brain that are the direct anatomico-physiological substrate of the maturation of the mathematical abilities adequate to age, without a simultaneous disorder of general mental functions.
> (Kosc, 1974, p. 47)

Butterworth further refines his definition by specifying that dyscalculia is a domain-specific core deficit in what he terms the "number module," which refers to the neurological structures that support processing and understanding of numbers (Butterworth, 2019). This is evident in the ability to comprehend numerosity, or the number of objects in a set, as well as the ability to compare number sets of different quantities, both of which are skills foundational to math development (Butterworth et al., 2011; Butterworth, 2019). Similarly, Knop and Chou (2020) define dyscalculia as a "core deficit in the approximate number system that allows subitizing (instant recognition of small quantities), estimation, and comparison of quantities" (p. 185), and Szucs et al. (2013) view dyscalculia as "a deficit of a core amodal magnitude representation often called 'number sense'" (p. 34). No matter the definition, researchers seem to be in agreement that dyscalculia is a biological, brain-based difference (Butterworth, 2019; DeFina & Moser, 2011; Knop & Chou, 2020; Szucs & Goswani, 2013).

The *Diagnostic and Statistical Manual of Mental Disorders*, 5th ed., commonly referred to as the DSM-5, refers to dyscalculia as a "specific learning disorder with impairment in math," and it is diagnosed based on persistent challenges in spite of interventions and in the absence of other underlying causes, including, among others, cognitive delays, physical disabilities, mental or neurological disorders, or lack of access (American Psychiatric Association, 2017). The World Health Organization's International Classification of Diseases, 10th ed. (ICD-10) similarly identifies dyscalculia as a "specific disorder of arithmetical skills" and bases diagnosis on "a specific impairment in arithmetical skills that is not solely explicable on the basis of general mental retardation or of inadequate schooling" (World Health Organization, 2009, as cited in Butterworth, 2019, p. 7). Further, the ICD-10 definition is specific to calculation and not other areas of math and excludes difficulties that may be compounded by comorbid conditions (Butterworth, 2019). While definitions vary, all share a consensus that dyscalculia is a biological, brain-based difference (Knop & Chou, 2020).

Diagnostic criteria for dyscalculia are not well established and vary among practitioners. As with other learning differences, identifying an achievement-IQ score discrepancy has been used to diagnose dyscalculia (Mazzocco & Myers, 2003), as well as low performance on math achievement tests (Butterworth et al., 2011). However, there are problems with these approaches, including lack of scientific evidence of their efficacy (Mazzocco & Myers, 2003). Persistent low achievement over time is also used as an indicator, but these individuals may not necessarily fit the criteria for dyscalculia (Geary, 1990). Furthermore, without a consensus on definitions, establishing agreed-upon diagnostic criteria is difficult, if not impossible. Mazzocco and Myers (2003) conducted research evaluating the effectiveness of different definitional criteria using persistent low achievement as a key indicator. Their results showed considerable inconsistency in ability to identify students with dyscalculia using a range of measures, which again points to the importance of establishing a consensus on definition and diagnostic criteria. In addition, it is difficult to determine effective strategies for remediation without a thorough understanding of the underlying cognitive basis of dyscalculia (Butterworth et al., 2011).

Subtypes of Dyscalculia

Researchers have identified different subtypes of dyscalculia, summarized in Table 2.1. Kosc (1974) identified six subtypes: verbal (difficulties with math language); practognostic (difficulties with manipulation of objects); lexical (difficulties reading math symbols); graphical (difficulties writing math symbols);

TABLE 2.1 Subtypes of dyscalculia

Subtype	Impact
Kosc (1974)	
Verbal	Math language
Practognostic	Manipulation of objects
Lexical	Reading math symbols
Graphical	Writing math symbols
Ideognostical	Understanding mathematical ideas
Operational development	Addition, subtraction, multiplication, and division
Geary (2004)	
Procedural	Verbal working memory
Semantic	Long-term memory retrieval
Visuospatial	Spatial representation of numbers
Feifer and Clark (2016)	
Procedural	Counting, ordering, and sequencing
Verbal	Identification of numbers and retrieval of facts
Semantic	Understanding magnitude
Von Aster (2000)	
Verbal	Counting, number identification, and retrieval of facts
Visual-Arabic	Number transcription, basic calculation, regrouping, and syntax
Semantic	Estimation, magnitude, and conceptual understanding

ideognostical (difficulties understanding mathematical ideas); and operational development (difficulties with addition, subtraction, multiplication, and division). Geary identified three subtypes: procedural, which may be related to verbal working memory deficits; semantic, which relates to long-term memory retrieval; and visuospatial, which refers to deficits in spatial representation of numbers (Geary, 2004; Mazzocco & Myers, 2003). Feifer and Clark (2016, as cited in Knop & Chou, 2020) also identified three subtypes: procedural, which is related to the ability to count, order, and sequence; verbal, which deals with identification of numbers and retrieval of facts; and semantic, which relates to understanding magnitude. Feifer and DeFina (2005, as cited in Knop & Cho, 2020) include a fourth subtype, visuospatial, with all four of these subtypes associated with specific regions of the brain. Von Aster (2000) also identifies subtypes that are linked to specific brain regions: verbal dyscalculia, which affects counting, number identification, and retrieval of facts; visual-Arabic dyscalculia, which affects number transcription, basic calculation, regrouping, and syntax; and semantic dyscalculia, which affects estimation, magnitude, and conceptual understanding. Researchers have different ways of classifying subtypes, though there is considerable overlap in their approaches.

A lack of research concerning strategies and support for individuals with dyscalculia leaves open the possibility that there may be, in addition to the subtypes, a form of the difference which could be considered a delay, rather than a cognitive deficit, and which could be overcome through appropriate intervention (Butterworth et al., 2011).

Cognitive Underpinnings/Neuroscience of Dyscalculia

While there is considerable disagreement about the definitions and nature of dyscalculia, researchers seem to be in agreement that it is a biological, brain-based learning difference (Butterworth, 2019; DeFina & Moser, 2011; Knop & Chou, 2020; Szucs & Goswani, 2013). However, complicating this understanding is neuroimaging evidence that shows mathematics is processed in multiple parts of the brain (DeFina & Moser, 2011; von Aster, 2000). Some studies suggest structural and functional differences in the brains of dyscalculics versus neurotypical individuals (Butterworth et al., 2011; Butterworth, 2019). Butterworth et al. (2011) cite multiple areas of the brain where structural and/or functional differences may be present, including reduced activation in the left and right intraparietal sulci (IPS), reduced gray matter density in areas of the brain associated with numerical processing, and reduced connectivity among regions of the parietal lobe, as well as between parietal and occipitotemporal regions that process symbolic numbers. Longitudinal studies show differences in the density of gray and white matter in dyscalculic brains (McCaskey et al., 2020). Butterworth's domain-specific core deficit theory points to structural and functional differences in the parietal lobe of children with dyscalculia (2019). Some dispute the core deficit theory and suggest that the heterogeneous nature of dyscalculia precludes this (Kaufmann et al., 2003). Others contend that dyscalculia is a result of a domain-general deficit in logical reasoning ability (Morsanyi et al., 2013). Szucs et al. (2013) present yet another alternative theory, which is that dyscalculia is related to visuospatial short-term memory and working memory.

Dyscalculia subtype models point to specific areas of the brain that are affected by dyscalculia (DeFina & Moser, 2011). For example, von Aster's (2000) verbal, visual-Arabic, and semantic subtypes point to deficits in the left perisylvian region, the bilateral occipital temporal lobes, and the bilateral inferior parietal lobes, respectively. Similarly, Feifer and DeFina's (2005) verbal, procedural, and semantic subtypes are related to these same areas, with the additional visuospatial subtype showing a connection to the bilateral occipital parietal lobes.

Complexities and Co-occurring Conditions

Math development and learning is complex (Dehaene, 2011; Geary, 2004; Karagiannakis et al., 2014). Unlike the development of reading skills, the development of math occurs along a trajectory throughout childhood and beyond, with different performance demands and changes in the skills required for understanding (Mazzocco & Myers, 2003). Math understanding involves multiple skills, including reasoning, working memory, language, and spatial cognition, and a deficit in any one of these areas can have a negative impact on math performance (Butterworth et al., 2011). Additionally,

> [M]athematics is a complex subject including different domains such as arithmetic, arithmetic problem solving, geometry, algebra, probability, statistics, calculus, . . . that implies mobilizing a variety of basic abilities associated with the sense of quantity, symbols decoding, memory, visuospatial capacity, logics, to name a few. Students with difficulties in any of these abilities or in their coordination, may experience mathematical learning difficulties.
> (Karagiannakis et al., 2014, **p. 1**)

This presents a challenge for uncovering the underlying mechanisms of dyscalculia. Adding to this complexity is the fact that multiple reasons besides dyscalculia can explain poor math achievement, such as domain-general factors that affect learning, math anxiety, lack of access to quality teaching, and other environmental factors, such as socioeconomic status and home life (Butterworth, 2019; Knop & Chou, 2020). Other learning differences, such as dyslexia, have also been noted for their negative impact on math (Mazzocco & Myers, 2003). The impact of working memory on math achievement, which is important for many mathematical tasks, is beginning to be understood (Allen et al., 2020; Allen et al., 2019; Friedman et al., 2018). Math anxiety is well researched and has been shown to have a significant impact on math achievement (Ashcraft & Krause, 2007; Furner & Berman, 2003; Herts & Beilock, 2017; Mutlu, 2019). Co-occurring conditions present a unique challenge due to the complexity of the interaction between multiple exceptionalities (Baum et al., 2017), and dyscalculia has been found to frequently occur alongside other learning differences, especially dyslexia (Butterworth et al., 2011).

Because math development is complex and math itself involves varied concepts, skills, and tasks, it's possible for students to perform well in some areas of math but struggle in others, further complicating a diagnosis (Gersten et al., 2005).

Twice Exceptional/2e

Growing research into twice exceptionality, or 2e, frames these learners through a strength-based, talent-focused lens (Baum et al., 1995; Baum et al., 2014; Baum & Schader, 2018; Olenchak, 2009; Reis et al., 2014). Therefore, this study will be placed in the context of twice exceptionality, in this case, gifted learners with dyscalculia. According to Reis et al. (2014) 2e individuals "demonstrate the potential for high achievement or creative productivity in one or more domains" and "manifest one or more disabilities." These traits "combine to produce a unique population of students who may fail to demonstrate either high academic performance or specific disabilities. Their gifts may mask their disabilities and their disabilities may mask their gifts" (Reis et al., 2014, p. 222).

Many students with dyscalculia are unidentified until problems begin around second or third grade; however, for gifted students, evidence of challenge for some may not be clear until middle school (Knop & Chou, 2020). Considering the neuroscience of dyscalculia in the context of 2e learners in general adds another layer of complexity for dyscalculic students.

> Teachers, for instance, often are confused by conflicting abilities in the same child, and parents often are unable to get services for their child because the child does not fit any clear diagnostic scheme or qualification criteria. More well-designed neuroscientific study of the gifted and [2e] would help ameliorate some of these difficulties.
> (Gilger & Hynd, 2008, p. 216)

There is scant research on dyscalculia among gifted students (Knop & Chou, 2020). It is possible for a student to experience difficulties associated with dyscalculia but fall within the average to superior range in mathematics due to giftedness or access to effective accommodations. Knop and Chou (2020) refer to this as "stealth dyscalculia," borrowing from the terminology for stealth dyslexia. These students may struggle with retrieval of facts and procedural knowledge but excel as a result of superior verbal reasoning, working memory, and/or fluid intelligence and, as a result, may not be identified until much later than is typical (Knop & Chou, 2020).

A strength-based, talent-focused approach with students demonstrating dual exceptionalities is an effective teaching practice (Baum et al., 2017). Research has shown multiple benefits of a strength-based approach, such as stronger social relationships with peers; improved ability to deal with social, emotional, and cognitive challenges; opportunities to form professional relationships with adults through mentoring; and development of expertise in talent areas (Baum et al., 2014). This approach has also been shown to increase both academic achievement and positive self-concept (Baum et al., 1995; Olenchak, 2009; Reis et al., 2014). In studies of 2e students, a focus on strengths and a de-emphasis on disability lead to students whose gifted characteristics are more apparent socially, emotionally, and academically and who are more engaged and able to be successful (Reis et al., 2014).

Research into different learning differences has provided opportunities to reframe these neurological differences as strengths to be recognized, nurtured, and celebrated. For example, children with ADHD are known to have strengths in logical reasoning, emotional intelligence, and creativity (Climie & Mastoras, 2015). They are also recognized for their strengths in divergent thinking and their ability to get into a "flow" state (Armstrong, 2010). Dyslexic students tend to be creative and excel at "big-picture" thinking (Schneps, 2014). They also have visual-spatial strengths, such as efficient perception of visual information and ease with 3D visualization and spatial problem solving (Armstrong, 2010; Rappolt-Schlichtmann et al., 2018). Eide and Eide (2012) have identified what they term MIND strengths in those with dyslexia. These strengths include material, interconnected, narrative, and dynamic reasoning. Individuals on the autism spectrum can be highly detail-oriented and systematic thinkers, which can lead to strengths in subjects that benefit from a systematic approach, such as math, science, and technology (Wright, 2013).

Strength-Based, Talent-Focused Lens of Dyscalculia

Much of the research on dyscalculia focuses on this learning difference through the medical model, solely as a deficit to be remediated. There is very little in the literature that places dyscalculia in a positive, strength-based light. Lewis and Lynn (2018) successfully reframe dyscalculia as a cognitive difference rather than a deficit in their study of a statistics major with dyscalculia. Their research brings up issues of accessibility for those who process math differently and the value of leveraging alternative tools and developing compensatory strategies. Lewis and Lynn also challenge myths associated with math ability, including the belief that those with dyscalculia are unable to learn higher-level math, and bring attention to what those with dyscalculia can do, as opposed to what they cannot do. Karagiannakis et al. (2014) have found that when working with students with dyscalculia, intervention that focuses on strengths can better support compensation for areas of deficit while also building motivation, whereas too much emphasis on deficits leads to decreased motivation and failure. There is further evidence that a focus on strengths, as filtered through multiple intelligences theory, yields higher academic achievement in math for students with dyscalculia (Al-Zoubi & Al-Adawi, 2019).

Literature Review Summary

This overview of the research literature provides a current understanding of the definitions and diagnostic criteria of dyscalculia, highlighting the lack of consensus on these issues, as well as differing views on possible subtypes of this learning difference.

In spite of that lack of consensus, literature related to the cognitive underpinnings of dyscalculia points to a widely held view of it as a biological, brain-based learning difference (Butterworth, 2019; DeFina & Moser, 2011; Knop & Chou, 2020; Szucs & Goswani, 2013) and demonstrates that multiple areas of the brain are involved. Co-occurring conditions and the complexities of math learning, including the multitude of reasons for lack of achievement in math, further point to challenges in understanding and diagnosing dyscalculia. Research related to twice-exceptionality and a strength-based, talent-focused approach to teaching and learning presents a rationale for placing this study in the context of twice exceptionality and demonstrates a gap in the literature concerning gifted individuals with dyscalculia. Finally, the vast majority of the research on dyscalculia follows a deficit model, and there is a significant gap in the literature that places dyscalculia in a strength-based light.

Dyscalculia is a poorly understood learning difference, with research lagging far behind that of other learning differences. Research in strength-based learning has shown positive outcomes for 2e learners; therefore, a strength-based lens of dyscalculia could advance understanding of this learning difference while laying a foundation for dyscalculia to be understood as a cognitive difference with a unique set of strengths to be developed, rather than solely as a problem to be fixed.

Positive Psychology

Merriam and Tisdell (2016) refer to the theoretical framework of a study as "the underlying structure, the scaffolding or frame" (p. 85) or as the "lenses" through which phenomena are studied (p. 85). It is through this lens that decisions are made with regard to the problem of the study, as well as research questions, methodology, and interpretation of the data (Merriam & Tisdell, 2016). The theoretical framework selected for this study is positive psychology.

Positive psychology, which grew from the work of Seligman and Csikszentmihalyi (2000), takes a holistic view of the individual by refocusing away from exclusive attention to deficits and toward understanding of strengths. Since World War II, the bulk of the work of psychology centered on identification, treatment, and prevention of diseases and problems (Pluskota, 2014; Seligman & Csikszentmihalyi, 2000). This approach, however, "ignored or denied those possibilities and potentials which could be realized through accessing underlying basic strengths" (Pluskota, 2014, p. 2). Positive psychology holds a research-supported view that a focus on recognizing and nurturing strengths can help an individual reach his or her potential.

> The aim of positive psychology is to begin to catalyze a change in the focus of psychology from preoccupation only with repairing the worst things in life to also building positive qualities.
> (Seligman & Csikszentmihalyi, 2000, **p. 5**)

This can also apply to education, in which a deficit view is often the lens through which teachers, educational psychologists, parents, and others approach students with learning differences. Studies support that when attention in schools is balanced between strengths and deficits, students can succeed (Baum et al., 1997; Olenchak, 1995). Positive psychology does not ignore the challenges associated with learning differences, but it suggests that a sole focus on deficits leads to an incomplete understanding of an individual's potential (Peterson, 2009).

> Ultimately, positive psychology offers a more balanced, holistic, and hopeful approach to a population typically viewed through a deficit lens and has the potential to inspire a greater emphasis on building capacity in these children and their families and schools.
> (Climie & Mastoras, 2015, **p. 296**)

When there is a balanced view of both problems and strengths, positive psychology allows for using what is identified as an asset to address what is identified as a deficit (Peterson, 2009).

Summary

Dyscalculia is a learning difference that is very much viewed through a deficit lens; however, as noted earlier, research into other learning differences is revealing that advantages can be associated with specific learning differences. In addition, using strengths to address deficits is an effective strategy for remediation and personal growth. Using positive psychology as a theoretical framework, this study seeks to reframe dyscalculia as a cognitive difference in which strengths can be recognized, nurtured, and leveraged as tools for success. "Treatment is not just fixing what is broken, it is nurturing what is best" (Seligman & Csikszentmihalyi, 2000, p. 7).

References

Allen, K., Giofrè, D., Higgins, S., & Adams, J. (2020). Working memory predictors of written mathematics in 7- to 8-year-old children. *The Quarterly Journal of Experimental Psychology*, 73(2), 239–248. https://doi.org/10.1177/1747021819871243

Allen, K., Higgins, S., & Adams, J. (2019). The relationship between visuospatial working memory and mathematical performance in school-aged children: A systematic review. *Educational Psychology Review*, 31(3), 509–531. https://doi.org/10.1007/s10648-019-09470-8

Al-Zoubi, S., & Al-Adawi. F. (2019). Effects of instructional activities based on Multiple Intelligences Theory on academic achievement of Omani students with dyscalculia. *Journal for the Education of Gifted Young Scientists*, 7(1), 1–25. https://files.eric.ed.gov/fulltext/ED606223.pdf

American Psychiatric Association. (2017). Neurodevelopmental disorders. In *Diagnostic and statistical manual of mental disorders* (5th ed., pp. 66–74). American Psychiatric Association Publishing. https://www.psychiatry.org/psychiatrists/practice/dsm

Armstrong, T. (2010). *The power of neurodiversity: Unleashing the advantages of your differently wired brain*. Da Capo Press. https://www.hachettebookgroup.com/titles/thomas-armstrong-phd/the-power-of-neurodiversity/9780738215242/?_ga=2.228764444.1609041706.1678893626-1451415088.1678893626

Ashcraft, M. H., & Krause, J. A. (2007). Working memory, math performance, and math anxiety. *Psychonomic Bulletin & Review, 14*(2), 243–248. https://link.springer.com/content/pdf/10.3758/BF03194059.pdf

Baum, S., Cooper, C., Neu, T., & Owen, S. (1997). *Evaluation of project High Hopes* (Project R206a30159-95). U.S. Department of Education.

Baum, S. M., Renzulli, J. S., & Hebert, T. P. (1995). Reversing underachievement: Creative productivity as a systematic intervention. *Gifted Child Quarterly, 39*(4), 224–235. https://doi.org/10.1177/001698629503900406

Baum, S. M., & Schader, R. (2018). Using a positive lens: Engaging twice exceptional learners. In S. B. Kaufman (Ed.), *Twice exceptional: Supporting and educating bright and creative students with learning difficulties* (pp. 48–65). Oxford Press. https://psycnet.apa.org/record/2018-09007-002

Baum, S. M., Schader, R., & Owen, S. (2017). *To be gifted and learning disabled: Strength-based strategies for helping twice-exceptional students with LD, ADHD, and more.* Prufrock Press. https://www.routledge.com/To-Be-Gifted-and-Learning-Disabled-Strength-Based-Strategies-for-Helping/Baum-Schader-Owen/p/book/9781618216441

Baum, S. M., Schader, R. M., & Hébert, T. P. (2014). Through a different lens. *Gifted Child Quarterly, 58*(4), 311–327. https://doi.org/10.1177/0016986214547632

Butterworth, B. (2019). *Dyscalculia: From science to education.* Routledge. https://www.routledge.com/Dyscalculia-from-Science-to-Education/Butterworth/p/book/9781138688612

Butterworth, B., Varma, S., & Laurillard, D. (2011). Dyscalculia: From brain to education. *Science, 332*(6033), 1049–1053. https://doi.org/10.1126/science.1201536

Climie, E. A., & Mastoras, S. M. (2015). ADHD in schools: Adopting a strengths-based perspective. *Canadian Psychology, 56*(3), 295–300. https://doi.org/10.1037/cap0000030

DeFina, P. A., & Moser, R. S. (2011). An overview of neuroscience contributions to the understanding of dyscalculia in children. In A. S. Andrew (Ed.), *Handbook of pediatric neuropsychology* (pp. 683–687). Springer. https://psycnet.apa.org/record/2010-23861-054

Dehaene, S. (2011). *The number sense: How the mind creates mathematics.* Oxford University Press. https://global.oup.com/academic/product/the-number-sense-9780199753871?q=The%20number%20sense&lang=en&cc=us

Eide, B., & Eide, F. (2012). *The dyslexic advantage: Unlocking the hidden potential of the dyslexic brain.* Penguin. https://www.penguinrandomhouse.com/books/713579/the-dyslexic-advantage-revised-ad-updated-by-brock-eide-md-ma-and-fernette-eide-md/

Feifer, S. G., & Clark, H. K. (2016). *FAM: Feifer assessment of mathematics.* PAR.

Feifer, S. G., & DeFina, P. A. (2005). *The neuropsychology of mathematics: Diagnosis and intervention.* Middletown, MD: School Neuropsych Press, LLC.

Friedman, L. M., Rapport, M. D., Orban, S. A., Eckrich, S. J., & Calub, C. A. (2018). Applied problem solving in children with ADHD: The mediating roles of working memory and mathematical calculation. *Journal of Abnormal Child Psychology, 46*(3), 491–504. https://doi.org/10.1007/s10802-017-0312-7

Furner, J. M., & Berman, B. T. (2003). Math anxiety: Overcoming a major obstacle to the improvement of student math performance. *Childhood Education, 79*(3), 170–174. https://doi.org/10.1080/00094056.2003.10522220

Geary, D. C. (1990). A componential analysis of an early learning deficit in mathematics. *Journal of Experimental Child Psychology, 49,* 363–383.

Geary, D. C. (2004). Mathematics and learning disabilities. *Journal of Learning Disabilities, 37*(1), 4–15. https://doi.org/10.1177/00222194040370010201

Gersten, R., Jordan, N. C., & Flojo, J. R. (2005). Early identification and interventions for students with mathematics difficulties. *Journal of Learning Disabilities, 38*(4), 293–304. https://doi.org/10.1177/00222194050380040301

Gilger, J. W., & Hynd, G. W. (2008). Neurodevelopmental variation as a framework for thinking about the twice exceptional. *Roeper Review, 30*(4), 214–228. https://doi.org/10.1080/02783190802363893

Herts, J. B., & Beilock, S. L. (2017). From Janet T. Spence's manifest anxiety scale to the present day: Exploring math anxiety and its relation to math achievement. *Sex Roles, 77*(11–12), 718–724. https://doi.org/10.1007/s11199-017-0845-9

Karagiannakis, G., Baccaglini-Frank, A., & Papadatos, Y. (2014). Mathematical learning difficulties subtypes classification. *Frontiers in Human Neuroscience, 8.* https://doi.org/10.3389/fnhum.2014.00057

Kaufmann, L., Handl, P., & Thöny, B. (2003). Evaluation of a numeracy intervention program focusing on basic numerical knowledge and conceptual knowledge: A pilot study. *Journal of Learning Disabilities, 36*(6), 564–573. https://doi.org/10.1177/00222194030360060701

Knop, N. F., & Chou, S. H. (2020). Giftedness and math difficulty. In C. M. Fugate, W. Behrens, & C. Boswell (Eds.), *Understanding twice exceptional learners: Connecting research to practice* (pp. 183–216). Prufrock Press. https://www.routledge.com/Understanding-Twice-Exceptional-Learners-Connecting-Research-to-Practice/Fugate-Behrens-Boswell/p/book/9781646320776

Kosc, L. (1974). Developmental dyscalculia. *Journal of Learning Disabilities, 7*(3), 164–177. https://journals.sagepub.com/doi/10.1177/002221947400700309

Lewis, K. E., & Lynn, D. M. (2018). Against the odds: Insights from a statistician with dyscalculia. *Education Sciences, 8*(2), 63–82. https://doi.org/10.3390/educsci8020063

Mazzocco, M. M., & Myers, G. F. (2003). Complexities in identifying and defining mathematics learning disability in the primary school-age years. *Annals of Dyslexia, 53*(1), 218–253. https://doi.org/10.1007/s11881-003-0011-7

McCaskey, U., von Aster, M., O'Gorman, R., & Kucian, K. (2020). Persistent differences in brain structure in developmental dyscalculia: A longitudinal morphometry study. *Frontiers in Human Neuroscience, 14*, 272. https://doi.org/10.3389/fnhum.2020.00272

Merriam, S. B., & Tisdell, E. J. (2016). *Qualitative research: A guide to design and implementation*. Jossey-Bass. https://www.wiley.com/en-us/Qualitative+Research:+A+Guide+to+Design+and+Implementation,+4th+Edition-p-9781119003618

Morsanyi, K., Devine, A., Nobes, A., & Szűcs, D. (2013). The link between logic, mathematics and imagination: Evidence from children with developmental dyscalculia and mathematically gifted children. *Developmental Science, 16*(4), 542–553. https://doi.org/10.1111/desc.12048

Mutlu, Y. (2019). Math anxiety in students with and without math learning difficulties. *International Electronic Journal of Elementary Education, 11*(5), 471–475. https://doi.org/10.26822/iejee.2019553343

Olenchak, F. R. (1995). Effects of enrichment on gifted/learning disabled students. *Journal for the Education of the Gifted, 18*, 385–399. https://journals.sagepub.com/doi/10.1177/016235329501800403

Olenchak, F. R. (2009). Effects of talents unlimited counseling on gifted/learning disabled students. *Gifted Education International, 25*(2), 144–164. https://doi.org/10.1177/026142940902500205

Peterson, C. (2009). Positive psychology. *Reclaiming Children and Youth, 18*(2), 3–7. https://eric.ed.gov/?id=EJ867919

Pluskota, A. (2014). The application of positive psychology in the practice of education. *SpringerPlus, 3*(1), Article 147. https://doi.org/10.1186/2193-1801-3-147

Rappolt-Schlichtmann, G., Boucher, A. R., & Evans, M. (2018). From deficit remediation to capacity building: Learning to enable rather than disable students with dyslexia. *Language, Speech & Hearing Services in Schools (Online), 49*(4), 864–874. https://doi.org/10.1044/2018_LSHSS-DYSLC-18-0031

Reis, S. M., Baum, S. M., & Burke, E. (2014). An operational definition of twice-exceptional learners: Implications and applications. *Gifted Child Quarterly, 58*, 217–230. https://journals.sagepub.com/doi/abs/10.1177/0016986214534976

Schneps, M. (2014). The advantages of dyslexia. *Scientific American Mind, 26*(1), 24–25. https://www.scientificamerican.com/article/the-advantages-of-dyslexia/

Seligman, M. E. P., & Csikszentmihalyi, M. (2000). Positive psychology: An introduction. *American Psychologist, 55*(1), 5–14. https://doi.org/10.1037/0003-066X.55.1.5

Szucs, D., Devine, A., Soltesz, F., Nobes, A., & Gabriel, F. (2013). Developmental dyscalculia is related to visuo-spatial memory and inhibition impairment. *Cortex, 49*(10), 2674–2688. https://doi.org/10.1016/j.cortex.2013.06.007

Szucs, D., & Goswani, U. (2013). Dyscalculia: Fresh perspectives. *Trends in Neuroscience and Education, 2*(2), 33–37. https://www.sciencedirect.com/science/article/pii/S2211949313000185

von Aster, M. (2000). Developmental cognitive neuropsychology of number processing and calculation: Varieties of developmental dyscalculia. *European Child & Adolescent Psychiatry, 9*(S2). https://doi.org/10.1007/s007870070008

Wright, A. (2013). *Academic and cognitive trends in children living with autism* (Proquest No. 1522778) [Master's thesis, California State University, Fullerton].

3

Profiles

The purpose of this study was to explore the strengths, experiences, and perceptions of gifted adults with dyscalculia. This chapter presents general profiles of the participants interviewed, including information about their background and demographics, hobbies and interests, diagnosis of dyscalculia and any co-occurring conditions descriptions of the impact of dyscalculia on their lives, evidence of their giftedness, identified strengths and opportunities to develop them, and insight about their self-concept and perceptions. An overview of the participants' demographics is presented in Table 3.1. The profiles are intended as an introduction to the participants and to provide context for their stories in the next chapter.

James

Background and Demographics
James is a 51-year-old white male living in the southeastern United States. He is married with no children. He is the fourth of five children in his family, and all of his siblings were academic high achievers and are now university professors. He is a college dropout and began working as a software developer while still in high school, running his own business by his early to mid-20s. James had an unusual childhood. He grew up in a

TABLE 3.1 Participant demographics

Pseudonym	Age at time of interview	Gender	Region of the United States	Age/grade at dyscalculia diagnosis
James	51	M	Southeastern	Grade 3
Emma	31	F	Pacific Northwest	26
Amelia	19	F	Pacific Coast	18
Sylvia	44	F	Upper Midwest	Grade 8
Louisa	26	F	New England	21

cult in California until his parents decided to leave when he was approximately in the third grade.

Hobbies and Interests

James is athletic and was involved in competitive bicycle racing in his youth. He has been deeply interested in computers beginning at a very young age. At the time of his interview, he was writing a book about his life experiences.

Dyscalculia Diagnosis and Co-occurring Conditions

James reports that the education system at the cult compound was similar to Montessori-based schools, and he was showing signs of struggle in math, reading, and writing even then. He was evaluated after moving away from the cult and was diagnosed in third grade as having dyslexia, dysgraphia, and "math dyslexia."

Impact of Dyscalculia

James describes his school experiences as "massively frustrating." In speaking about his struggles, specifically with trying to learn and master multiplication tables, he notes that his difficulties made him think there was "a level of stupid" he must be, and he was surprised and confused by his inability to learn math facts. He had always been behind his peers academically, even while in the alternative school system of the cult. After his initial diagnosis, James was moved to a school he describes as a magnet school for students with learning disabilities, and he participated in special education programs from that point through high school. He explains that a lot of teachers put a lot of effort into teaching him math, but he had a "profound" inability to learn. He notes that his frustration sometimes caused him to stop trying, but that in general he tried very hard to succeed and is still surprised by his inability to do math, especially in light of his work in a field that is so often connected to math. He sees the efforts by himself and his teachers as a "huge amount of wasted time." He feels the only benefit of his special education experience was that he was exempt from certain required classes and was still able to graduate high school. James feels a lot of anger about the trauma of his educational experiences and has strong negative opinions about the education system in general.

James was allowed to attend college on a provisional basis because he was missing math credits. He was at a considerable disadvantage because he was so "hopelessly behind on math, because I hadn't done anything, any math-related work, and math was now a requirement." He even struggled in his computer science classes, which he felt should have been manageable as he was already working as a software developer; however, because those classes had a "mathematical-oriented approach to computers," he was unable to be successful and failed every computer science class he tried to take. Being so far behind led to failing grades, academic suspension, and then dropping out after three semesters.

As an adult, James doesn't feel his dyscalculia negatively affects his life in any major way, saying that feels he experiences "zero problems" as an adult as a result of dyscalculia. He does go on to say, however, that he has confidence issues stemming from his learning differences, still needs to use his fingers to calculate even single-digit numbers, and has trouble with scheduling and budgeting. In spite of these challenges, James believes that his coping mechanisms prevent those issues from being significant roadblocks in his daily life.

Evidence of Giftedness

James is an articulate person with a strong command of language and a depth of self-awareness. His above-average ability in computers is evidenced by his acquisition of a software patent in his 20s and through recognition by his peers, who call him "professor" for his command of computer knowledge. Also, as noted earlier, James was running his own software development business by his early 20s.

Strengths

James points to his strengths as working with computers (especially software design), as well as perseverance, creativity (especially lateral thinking), oral communication, and writing. James also recognizes that he has strong people skills in certain contexts, especially in his work environment.

While in high school, James had the opportunity to join an AP computer science class. At that time, the teacher of the class recognized that his skills and understanding far outpaced her own. He describes that experience as being boring because the pacing of the class was too slow for his abilities and needs. The teacher allowed him to work at his own pace, move ahead in the textbook, and complete projects out of the textbook on his own. Soon after, he was recommended for an internship program, which he described as "groundbreaking" and notes that this experience allowed him to escape the label as a student with learning differences because the adults at his internship were unaware of his academic struggles and only saw him as an intern who performed his job well. Due to his success and high ability in that internship, he was able to parlay it into a paying job while still in high school.

Self-Concept/Perception

According to James, "Struggles with academia have been the defining thing in my life," and he wonders whether his experiences in special education did him more harm than good. He recognizes the irony of having dyscalculia and being so successful in his field, noting that a lot of people wouldn't believe that someone could be so profoundly bad at math and be a software developer. James also laments that dyscalculia doesn't have the same level of awareness and acceptance as dyslexia. He struggles to understand it himself: "It just doesn't make any sense that I can't do those things."

Emma

Background and Demographics
Emma is a 31-year-old white female college graduate living with her husband in the Pacific Northwest. She has no children, but takes in foster children from time to time. She was pursuing a master's degree in counseling psychology, but has opted to take time off to focus on her artistic and writing strengths by writing and illustrating a children's book. Emma has been active in paid and volunteer work helping trafficked women and children, a cause for which she has a strong passion.

Hobbies and Interests
Emma has many creative interests. She is a writer and visual artist. She is also musically inclined and is a self-taught musician on guitar, ukulele, piano, violin, banjo, and cello. As evidenced by her now-paused pursuit of a master's degree in psychology, Emma is very interested in people. Emma also enjoys spending time outdoors in nature, especially birdwatching and sketching.

Dyscalculia Diagnosis and Co-occurring Conditions
Emma was not diagnosed with dyscalculia until she was 26 years old. She pursued neuropsychological testing after recognizing characteristics of herself in a description of dyscalculia while researching individualized education program (IEP) accommodations for a five-year-old foster child. According to Emma,

> Specifically, there was one instance where we were sitting there, and we were having . . . lunch, and I was helping him do his math worksheet and I said, "Oh, this is two plus two is six," or I didn't know, I said the wrong thing. And my five-year-old said, "No, mommy, it's this," and he said the correct thing, and I [realized] even these basic math skills are really lacking for me. And [there were] just little things like that over time. And then, when I was advocating for my son getting an IEP and different things to support him in school so that he

could actually thrive in school, I was scrolling through this list of disabilities to see how he could get his assessments and everything. And I saw dyscalculia, math learning disability. I didn't think that he had that, but I was like, "Oh my gosh, there's a math learning disability?" Like, what? And so I googled it, and looked it all up, and everything was me. I literally just started crying, and I was like, "Oh my gosh, this is me."

Impact of Dyscalculia

Emma struggled greatly with math throughout her schooling and life. She describes herself as being "bad at numbers" and having "a whole slew" of things that she now recognizes as being related to dyscalculia. She noticed she struggled with things like "I don't know my left from my right, [and other] typical dyscalculia things regarding time, and how many times it took me to pass my driver's license test, so many things that now I know they're dyscalculia related." She was a high academic achiever in school and is honest about resorting to cheating at times to get through math classes, both in high school and in college. Looking back, Emma believes her gaps in math throughout her schooling were chalked up to the unstable home life of being a child growing up in the foster care system, and her strengths allowed her to compensate enough to be successful in school.

From an early age, Emma noticed that she struggled with things that seemed easier for her peers. She struggled with numbers and math, but the two challenges she remembers standing out the most from her early schooling were noticing that her peers seemed to understand time and what she now knows as subitizing, concepts that she was unable to grasp. She remembers being confused about what time it was and not understanding how other students knew those things. With regard to subitizing, she recognized that other students innately knew how many objects were in a group and knew how many objects were needed to pair them up, but she would "just grab things that made no sense" to the number of items needed. In describing her dyscalculia, Emma used language as an analogy and explained that math is like a foreign language that she cannot "learn or know or understand or comprehend."

Emma's math struggles in school were recognized, but as noted earlier, she believes the school attributed them to being the result of her unstable home life. To support her, she was offered tutoring, which she hated and found largely ineffective. She remembers tutoring as tedious and frustrating, and it amounted to just giving her more work to do. She did recognize, however, that being able to use manipulatives was somewhat helpful, a strategy she has carried into adulthood.

Dyscalculia presented a struggle in college as well, and not just in math classes but also in science classes and in any class where numbers were involved. She described a paper she wrote for a history class where the feedback from the professor was very complimentary about her writing, but he was confused as to why the dates she noted were wrong, having put "1589" instead of "1959," for example. In classes where she struggled, Emma spoke of having to "fudge" her way through and, as noted earlier, she did occasionally resort to cheating to get through math classes.

In her adult life, Emma sees dyscalculia as causing significant challenges. In cooking and baking, Emma is unable to use measuring cups and spoons, because she doesn't understand the fractions, and she has to work extra hard to understand and set the right oven temperature and know how long to cook or bake something. It took her multiple tries to pass the test for a driver's license. She also struggles with directions, including knowing left from right, and finds using a global positioning system (GPS) or maps to be unhelpful. Understanding speed limits is also a struggle, because she is not able to locate the number that is on the speed sign within the numerals shown on her speedometer. Time management is also a significant challenge, including gauging the length of time required to do a task and scheduling appointments. Emma provided an example of a struggle with time when she scheduled a dentist appointment and then scheduled an acupuncture appointment for 15 minutes later, not recognizing that 15 minutes didn't allow enough time to have the first appointment and then get to the second one.

Evidence of Giftedness

The assessment Emma had done at age 26 also identified her as gifted with strengths in writing, verbal comprehension, visual-spatial skills, and reasoning. In spite of her significant challenges, Emma graduated high school with 4.0 GPA and was valedictorian of her graduating class. She attributes these achievements to her strengths compensating for her weaknesses.

Strengths

Emma has many strengths, including writing, creativity (especially music and visual arts), and the strength areas noted in her neuropsychological testing results discussed previously. Emma also has a strong sense of empathy and well-developed interpersonal skills, noting that peers have referred to her as "the people whisperer."

Emma attended a Christian school with limited funding and few resources, so aside from her academic successes, Emma's strengths and talents were not recognized or developed in school. Taking time off from her graduate program is allowing her to put time and effort into developing those strengths that were not cultivated at a younger age, especially writing and art.

Self-Concept/Perception

In reflecting on her duality, Emma notes that she tends to minimize her giftedness and doesn't know how to reconcile the two halves of her. She says, "I haven't really known how to put those pieces together or what to do with that as an adult. [It] kind of feels disjointed and split apart." Emma is curious about what she may have missed out on by her late diagnosis and identification as 2e. She is also frustrated by the lack of awareness of and understanding about dyscalculia, which makes it difficult to advocate for herself, though she is becoming more open to it.

Amelia

Background and Demographics

Amelia is a 19-year-old white Hispanic female. She is a recent high school graduate living with her parents in the Pacific Coast region. She works as a server in a restaurant and assists a realtor and, at the time of the interview, was about to begin community college. She is the third of four sisters in her family, and while depression is something the sisters share in common, none of her siblings have been identified as having learning differences or giftedness. Amelia does note that her sisters have not been tested for giftedness, and she "would not be surprised" if they qualified.

Hobbies and Interests

Amelia's varied interests point to her creativity and love of hands-on work. She occupies herself with a variety of arts and crafts, including crochet, knitting, wax seals, water coloring, and baking. She is musically inclined and is self-taught on piano and guitar. She especially enjoys singing. She loves reading, especially mystery stories. She also enjoys making people happy by gifting them with things she has made. Recently, Amelia has added going to the gym to her list of hobbies.

Dyscalculia Diagnosis and Co-occurring Conditions

Amelia was diagnosed with attention deficit hyperactivity disorder (ADHD) while in eighth grade. While she began showing signs of struggle in math from an early age, Amelia was not formally diagnosed with dyscalculia until her senior year in high school. At this time, her earlier diagnosis of ADHD was confirmed, and she was also diagnosed with autism spectrum disorder and identified as gifted and, therefore, twice exceptional.

Amelia was not surprised by her diagnoses of dyscalculia and autism, but was caught off guard by the identification as gifted. She has since come to understand, aided by the psychologist who administered her testing, that her deficits masked her talents. As she put it, "I struggled so much in certain aspects, that the ones that I was really good at just kind of got muddled out."

Impact of Dyscalculia

Amelia remembers math as being a source of intense stress in school, saying that math had "always been difficult" and that she always felt "clueless." She remembers intense emotional distress related to her efforts in math class and struggled to explain to her teachers where her understanding was breaking down. She goes on to say that she's always felt embarrassed in math because she was unable to understand the material and felt stupid, and she was often "on the verge of tears" during math tests. She describes math classes as going through a repeating "heartbreaking cycle" of not understanding and crying and the frustration of having the class move on to the next unit just as she felt she might be beginning to catch on. Amelia explained that she tried very hard to learn but was unsuccessful.

Even though her math scores were very low on the assessment in eighth grade that resulted in her ADHD diagnosis, nothing was done to identify or support her math challenges. Once she was in high school, however, she did receive help through math tutoring, first from her older sisters and then from a cousin. In her later high school years, she received help from a tutoring center, where the director recognized characteristics of dyscalculia.

In her adult life, Amelia points to a few challenges she notices as a result of her dyscalculia. She has difficulty reading analog clocks, doesn't know how to read large numbers, struggles with adding and subtracting money, can't do simple calculations in her head, and still relies on counting on her fingers. Amelia still lives at home with her parents, so she is not yet independent and therefore hasn't yet had the opportunity to discover in what other ways having dyscalculia may affect her in adulthood.

Evidence of Giftedness

As noted earlier, Amelia was surprised by her identification as twice exceptional and had not previously been recognized, by herself or anyone else, as having high potential in any area. The scores on her neuropsychological evaluation, administered by a psychologist with experience in identifying twice exceptionality, showed superior or very superior scores in many areas, including the general abilities index (especially verbal comprehension, visual/spatial reasoning, and fluid reasoning); perceptual reasoning; grammar and mechanics; social context awareness (especially awareness of social cues and perspective taking); and vocabulary. The assessment results also indicated significant strengths in interpersonal skills, compassion, sense of humor, imagination, and integrity.

Strengths

Although Amelia is just beginning to recognize her strengths, she has many, including language, creativity (especially related to arts and music, but also problem solving), people skills, and leadership. Amelia sees herself as empathetic, reliable, a quick learner, and as having an ability to give attention to detail. Amelia is also fluent in Spanish.

Because Amelia's strengths were masked by her challenges throughout her schooling and she wasn't recognized as having high ability, she did not have many opportunities to develop her strengths. However, she was active in musical theater in middle school and participated in an Afro-Haitian dance class for two years in high school in which she excelled and became a leader.

Self-Concept/Perception

Amelia is still surprised by being identified as someone with giftedness. She had no recognition of or opportunity to develop her strengths, and she has difficulty recognizing how she can be gifted. She feels cheated by an education system that did not help her grow: "I feel like the educational system I grew up in did not help me grow as a person because it wasn't catered to my specific needs or how I was wired. So I kind of feel cheated from that."

Sylvia

Background and Demographics

Sylvia is a 44-year-old white elementary school social worker with a master's degree in social work. She is single and lives in the Upper Midwest region of the United States with her dogs.

Hobbies and Interests

Sylvia's interests reflect her love of the outdoors and nature. She enjoys hiking, kayaking, and biking. She is also, as her career would indicate, very interested in people. She is a keen observer of people and is fascinated by human nature.

Dyscalculia Diagnosis and Co-occurring Conditions

Sylvia's struggles with math presented at a young age; however, because her discrepant results were misinterpreted as averaging out, she was not formally diagnosed with dyscalculia until around eighth grade. In her early years, when seeking answers for her math problems, Sylvia received some testing; however, her parents were told at the time that her extreme scores (very low in math and very high in other areas) meant that she would eventually "even out."

Sylvia's eventual diagnosis came due to the efforts and advocacy of her mother, who worked hard over an extended period of time to get Sylvia's school to evaluate her and take her math difficulties more seriously. According to Sylvia, the school was reluctant to consider any actions that would place an otherwise bright student in special education, "guilting" her mother with comments like "You don't want to put her in a classroom with those kinds of kids."

When Sylvia's school finally relented and tested her using grade-level math assessments, she wasn't able to get past the second-grade content as a middle school student. Because she was more than three years delayed, the school allowed her to receive special education services for math.

Sylvia was recognized for her high potential and intelligence and tested for the gifted program around fourth or fifth grade; unfortunately, she did not make the cut for the program due to her low math scores. Sylvia also struggled with high anxiety throughout her childhood but was not diagnosed with anxiety until her college years.

Impact of Dyscalculia

Sylvia describes her experiences in math growing up as "horrible," adding that she wanted very much to succeed, and worked hard to do so, but was unable to make progress. Sylvia's mother worked with her at home and was concerned by her inability to retain information related to numbers and math. Sylvia recalls her mother saying,

> "You would get it, you would know the answer, and then I'd show you the same flashcard two minutes later and you wouldn't have a clue what the answer was." And my mother said, "That's when I started to wonder if you had, like brain damage, caused by an injury."

Once Sylvia was diagnosed with dyscalculia, she was moved to special education math classes, which continued through high school. At one point, she received Orton Gillingham tutoring outside of school. According to Sylvia, the tutoring wasn't helpful in supporting her math learning but did help her to develop better organizational skills.

At school Sylvia remembers struggling to get through math classes and relying on strategies not to learn, but just to help her get through the hour, such as avoiding work by going to the bathroom or pretending to know what was happening in class. She was constantly worried about being called on to answer a question or participate in some way. Sylvia spoke more about the high anxiety caused by math struggles, saying that her anxiety increased to the point that she was experiencing frequent panic attacks and had stopped eating. She tried hard to use her strengths to cover for her deficits but felt like a fake and an imposter.

Getting into college was a challenge due to her diagnosis, special education coursework, and the "creative scheduling" that her school allowed in order for her to be able to graduate. She visited 16 different colleges and spoke with people in the offices of students with disabilities. She said "We had some colleges laugh when they looked at my transcript and say, 'We would never.'" Ironically, at one of the colleges, she and her parents were "wined and dined" on the tour due to her success with her published book of poetry. Her hotel was paid for, and they invited her to speak to students in the writing program; however, when she went to the admissions office and handed them her transcript, she was rudely told, "I'm sorry, but if this were handed to us, we'd be throwing it in the trash can. We would never accept a student with these classes and scores."

Sylvia notes a number of ways that dyscalculia negatively affects her adult life. She is highly dependent on her mother for support with budgeting and managing her finances. She reports that time management and planning her schedule are difficult, noting that she doesn't fully comprehend "clock time" and is never sure how long a task should take. Cooking is a challenge because she struggles with understanding quantity and volume. Difficulties understanding measurement present challenges in many ways, including online shopping, where she struggles to understand and visualize the sizes listed for an item. Sylvia notes that problems due to dyscalculia sometimes show up in unexpected ways. For example, she struggles with finding her gate at an airport because she doesn't know where to find her gate number within the range of gates displayed on the signs.

Sylvia also talked about the impact of her math struggles on her relationships, both in childhood and as an adult. With regard to peer relationships growing up, she says she already struggled socially due to being an introvert, but her problems in math made her worry about her peers discovering her limitations with math. Her math difficulties also affected her relationship with her parents, which affected her identity development. She expressed that having to rely on her parents beyond what would be expected at a certain age shaped the way she sees herself. In her dating life, dyscalculia has presented a challenge because she sees that her limitations put additional responsibilities on a partner, and not all partners understand dyscalculia or have empathy for her challenges, which can result in conflict.

Evidence of Giftedness

Sylvia's mother and some teachers saw signs of her giftedness from an early age, particularly in her advanced reading comprehension, her ability to articulate her understanding of complex ideas, and the content of her writing. With the support of her mother and a teacher who recognized her gift for writing, Sylvia published a book of poetry when she was in middle school. Later, in college, when she recognized that her experiences might have value for others, she wrote and published a memoir.

Strengths

Sylvia's most obvious strengths are her writing ability. However, she also demonstrates multiple other strengths, many of which are relevant in her work as a social worker. She is articulate and, as expected due to her writing strengths, she has a strong command of language. She has strong interpersonal skills. She is empathetic, a strong listener, and a communicator. She is flexible and a strong creative problem solver, which serves her well in her work as well as in her strategies to cover for her deficits. Sylvia also has well-developed leadership skills.

Sylvia was fortunate to have a strong advocate in her mother, which led to multiple opportunities throughout her schooling to develop her strengths. In addition to the poetry book she wrote and published in middle school, Sylvia participated in high school theater productions, attended a summer camp for talented writers, and was dual enrolled in a college-level poetry class while in high school. She worked as a counselor at a summer camp, which she attributes to her eventual career path. Sylvia said the speaking tours for her memoir were an opportunity to develop her public speaking and communication skills. According to Sylvia, her participation in the Odyssey of the Mind program from elementary into middle school was one of the most important opportunities to develop her strengths. She referred to this as a "game changer." Her participation in this program built her confidence, allowed her to develop her creative problem-solving strengths, helped her to see that individuals have unique strengths, and gave her the opportunity to finally connect with like-minded peers.

Self-Concept/Perception

Sylvia realizes that she has the duality of being both gifted and having dyscalculia. She shared:

> It's always left me feeling like I walk in two worlds. And so I think that's the biggest impression that I have for my

identity and myself is that . . . I have these two extremes . . . I just never feel like I'm completely blended.

Sylvia also struggles with the extremes of her situation, noting, "I often feel like I have these two extremes that are always weighing on me, you know, and I never quite go as high as I could go and I never quite go as low as I could go."

Louisa

Background
Louisa is a 26-year-old white female who lives with her parents in New England. She is a high school graduate with some community college credits and at the time of her interviews was unemployed but working toward supporting herself as a full-time artist.

Hobbies and Interests
Louisa has a variety of interests, many of which are creative in nature or involve helping others. She is a digital artist, she writes poetry, she enjoys music and dance, and she has been active in advocacy for youth, people with disabilities, and the LGBTQ community. She also enjoys yoga and meditation.

Dyscalculia Diagnosis and Co-occurring Conditions
Louisa sees herself through the lens of three types of disabilities: physical, learning differences, and psychiatric. She has cerebral palsy; been diagnosed with dyscalculia; been identified as having deficits in working memory and processing speed; and experienced mental health struggles, including bipolar disorder, anxiety, eating disorders, and borderline personality disorder.

Louisa's struggles in math were recognized as early as first grade, and she received psychoeducational testing about every four years to monitor her progress. Although a high school psychologist identified her as twice exceptional at age 16 due to the discrepancies and extremes in her testing, she was not formally diagnosed with dyscalculia until she was 21 years old. After taking some community college courses and when considering going to college to pursue a degree, Louisa's mother decided a reevaluation was necessary, because, "She can't do math in college. She'll fail."

Impact of Dyscalculia

Due to cerebral palsy, Louisa started kindergarten with an IEP already in place:

> Because I had a physical disability, I think that made it easier for people to sort of spot some signs of learning difficulties, because I had a lot of one-on-one attention and interaction with special ed. professionals. . . . And my dyscalculia symptoms were and still are very severe.

In talking about how she felt about her math struggles from an early age, Louisa noted that she had no problem with anything related to literacy but couldn't understand math and was "really confused as to why it was confusing." Like Emma, Louisa also offered an analogy of math as a foreign language that everyone else seemed to understand but she could not. In speaking about the experience of struggling so much with math while excelling in other areas, Louisa explained that she felt like an "idiot" and sensed a "weird cognitive dissonance" because she felt "smart and stupid at the same time."

In spite of the obvious struggles she was having, repeatedly failing in her math work, teachers initially thought she would eventually "catch up." She was pulled occasionally for more intensive instruction at some point during first grade, and then was taken completely out of the regular class for special education math instruction during second grade. She continued to receive special ed. pull-out instruction for math through her third year of high school. Louisa feels that the extra support she received was helpful and was the reason why she was able to get through math in school, saying that without that support, she believes she would have "drowned" and failed every math class.

After her third year of high school, Louisa was transferred to a psychotherapeutic boarding school to repeat her junior year.

She remained at that school for her senior year and stayed on for a few years after graduation to receive more mental health support. She had not yet received a formal diagnosis at the time she transferred, and the boarding school did not follow her previous high school's support for math. Instead, she was placed in regular math classes, where the school said, "this is a smart kid and she's not trying hard enough. She's lazy."

Speaking about her experiences at the boarding school, Louisa shared that she worked hard to be successful but felt a lot of anger and frustration. She would go to class with a ready-to-work-hard attitude, would quickly get confused, and would then ask for help. She explained that the school just did not know how to help her and did not realize that she needed to be taught math differently. All she remembered the school offering was impatience and a directive to try harder to do the work without help and not being understood for who she was:

> When I didn't understand something, they were like, "You need to do this, you need to try this on your own." I just felt so furious . . . and it was so ironic, too, because this was supposed to be a special education school, but I think because it was psychiatric in nature, they thought it was a mental willpower thing. Whereas when I was at the general school, I feel like they saw the big picture, like this is a smart kid with physical and learning and psychiatric disabilities. They saw the intersection of gifted and three types of disabilities. I felt like at boarding school they didn't really see, and it was really confusing, like, "Why aren't you seeing this?"

Louisa feels a great deal of frustration around the fact that her math problems were recognized and she was being given support, but she was given no name for it until she was 21 years old. Her desire was to be able to say "flat out" that she had a learning disability in math, and she still feels frustrated that when she tried to claim that label for herself without a formal diagnosis, others interpreted that as "lying, or self-diagnosing," though it was clear that she had dyscalculia. The analogy she gives is,

> It was apparent that there was a problem . . . when I was eight, but no one gave it a name until I was 21. But I was, like, I swear I have dyscalculia because . . . I like to think of it [as] sort of like if someone had been for the past decade [getting] intermittently really sad . . . and they don't feel like doing anything, and they feel hopeless, and they're not sleeping. So you read a report like that for years, but no one actually says, this person has depression. They obviously do. They're basically talking about what depression is without actually saying it.

When Louisa took community college classes, her experiences with math went "horribly." She describes a situation that was very similar to her boarding school experiences, with teachers telling her to "try harder." She explains that she didn't start out being lazy, but after so much time asking for help and getting none, she began to put less effort into her work. In the end, she barely passed her exams, "didn't synthesize information," and used memorization and recall as much as she could to give correct answers "without really grasping the information."

After receiving a diagnosis, Louisa says the response from the boarding school, "was much different . . . they were much more validating. And one woman was like, 'Well, I'm happy that you can have accommodations,'" a response she finds ludicrous in light of the frustration she experienced and the clear need for support that wasn't received.

In her adult life, Louisa identifies a few challenges that result from having dyscalculia. She is unable to read analog clocks, struggles both physically and cognitively to handle cash and make change, and has difficulty understanding measurements, direction, and distance. Louisa has her own apartment and pays her own rent and bills; however, her parents are currently living with her to provide support for the tasks of daily living due to her cerebral palsy. Though she has plans and hopes to become more independent in the future, she is not fully independent and therefore hasn't yet had the opportunity to discover in what other ways having dyscalculia may affect her in adulthood.

Evidence of Giftedness

In spite of not being formally identified as gifted, except for the informal 2e label from her high school psychologist, Louisa's experiences demonstrate evidence of high ability and high potential in multiple domains. She received a departmental award in high school in recognition of excellence in writing, had a poem published in adulthood, and at the time of her interview was preparing for a public exhibition of her art. Louisa is highly articulate, with a sophisticated and rich vocabulary. She demonstrates a depth of self-awareness and ability to use creative analogies to express her thinking and experiences. Additionally, the results from Louisa's multiple testing experiences throughout her schooling pointed to many strengths, particularly in verbal comprehension and abstract verbal reasoning.

Strengths

Louisa is highly creative, with strengths in divergent thinking, for which she attributes her ability to write poetry and make connections between seemingly unrelated things. Louisa has also demonstrated leadership skills in her advocacy work, including participation in disability leadership conferences.

Though Louisa was not formally identified as gifted in school, she had multiple opportunities to develop her strengths and interests. She had classes in photography and graphic design, and she participated in poetry workshops. She was also active in her school choir for a few years in middle and high school, participated in regional music festivals, and was active in school musicals for a number of years from middle through high school. Louisa also participated in dance festivals, performing modern dance and ballet with a choreographer who had experience in working with dancers with cerebral palsy.

Self-Concept/Perception

In reflecting on her multiple identities of gifted, physically disabled, having learning differences, and mental health challenges, Louisa describes having a confused sense of self: "I'm so smart, . . . why can't I do that? And so I just have this very disoriented sort of self-perception in regards to my intelligence."

Louisa also expressed frustration about the lack of recognition for the experiences of people with dyscalculia, especially in twice-exceptional populations, in spite of the wealth of information about 2e individuals with other non-math learning differences.

Conclusion

The brief participant introductions presented in this chapter provide essential context for the next chapter, where the focus transitions from individual profiles to a deeper exploration of themes. Each participant contributes a distinct perspective shaped by their own unique experiences; however, patterns and shared experiences emerged across their rich and varied stories. Carrying these profiles forward will help readers connect more meaningfully with the exploration that follows.

4

Themes and Stories

The themes that emerge from the participants' stories reflect the complex and often contradictory realities of being a gifted adult with dyscalculia. Their experiences reveal how high intellectual potential can coexist with profound challenges, particularly in environments that fail to recognize, understand, or adequately support twice-exceptional learners. While each participant's story is shaped by unique factors—such as family background, diagnosis, and personal experiences—many of their experiences overlap and connect in meaningful ways: early and persistent academic struggles, the emotional toll of unmet needs, and a continuing effort to reconcile their giftedness with their challenges. By examining both the uniqueness of individual experiences and the patterns that emerge across them, a more nuanced and holistic understanding of giftedness and dyscalculia begins to take shape—one that challenges deficit-based models and underscores the need for responsive, strength-based approaches in both research and education.

Themes

Six major themes emerged from the interviews, including strengths of adults with dyscalculia, opportunities to develop strengths and interests, support received during schooling,

DOI: 10.4324/9781003527800-4

emotional and behavioral responses, math struggles, and strategies for navigating adult challenges.

Strengths of Adults With Dyscalculia

Each participant was unique in their experiences; however, commonalities were noted among them with regard to strengths, the way they leveraged their strengths, and the interests in which they engaged. In particular, there was a pattern of high ability in language skills, interpersonal skills, and creativity.

Language Skills

In education, many students often think of themselves as being a "math person" or a "language person." With the participants in this study, that anecdote seemed to hold true. All participants had strong evidence of high ability in language skills, both in writing and oral communication.

Four of the five participants were writers. James and Emma were writing books at the time of their interviews, Sylvia had published two books, and Louisa had won awards for her writing and had a poem published.

In speaking about her school experiences, Sylvia noted, "I was pretty good with anything having to do with language arts . . . in particular creative writing." As an eighth-grade student, Sylvia wrote and published a book of poetry, which garnered a lot of attention.

> I think at that point, maybe the book was in like a manuscript form of some kind, but we ended up self-publishing it. At first, we thought we'd be just living with 3,000 copies in our living room, [but] we sold out within the first three months, so it was like a local phenomenon. And then from there, the book got picked up by a national publisher, and then kind of took off.

The success of her earlier work, and the impact of her story on audiences during her speaking tours, prompted Sylvia to write a memoir in her mid-20s while in college: "And then in college . . . I decided to write a memoir . . . because I saw the power that it had to share your story. I couldn't believe the changes people felt . . . when they'd heard the story."

For Emma, when asked about strengths in school, she identified "definitely writing," adding, "I don't know how many teachers were, like, you should be an author, you should write books. My writing was off the charts." Emma further explained that in the face of her math struggles at school, she put all of her energy into writing: "I think in order to compensate, because . . . I'm really, really bad at math, so I would pour all of my time and effort into anything involving writing, reading."

When asked to elaborate on her strengths in writing, Louisa shared, "I got an award from my high school English department and it wasn't any piece of writing in particular, it . . . gave me recognition for excellent writing" and added that she had recently had a poem published. In reflecting on her experiences with her language strengths throughout her schooling, she noted that just as she had always struggled with math, she had always done well with language arts, stating, "I did great in English all throughout my schooling, from early elementary school all the way to late high school. I usually received As in English. I did really well on standardized English exams." She recognized her talent for language arts as early as in kindergarten literacy lessons and summed up her strengths in this subject by simply stating: "I aced that."

For James, reading and writing were difficult due to having dyslexia and dysgraphia, but he felt that "My coping strategies [included] . . . learning how to write well." He spoke about a memoir he was in the process of writing and feels that an ability to express himself in writing is a strength. He added that one way in which he developed and used his writing skills was by "arguing with people on the internet, because . . . you can enter into writing contests with people all the time."

While Amelia doesn't recognize writing as a strength for her, her neuropsychological evaluation indicated superior to very superior ability in grammar, writing mechanics, and spelling, and she takes pride in her strong vocabulary:

> I don't remember being good at a certain thing, but little things I didn't notice . . . whenever I read books, I like using all the new words I learned [in the book] . . . I think it's really boring to use the same words over and over again to explain things, when there are words that could explain it in such intense detail.

In addition to written language skills, many participants demonstrated strengths in oral communication. In their interviews, all of the participants came across as highly articulate and were able to express themselves thoughtfully, clearly, and with insight. This was a strength that many recognized in themselves.

James understood that his struggles and academic history would have made it very difficult to get a job, saying: "There was no way that I was going to be able to . . . [complete] a job application on paper. I would not have been hired for any job. But I could speak well and I could write software."

Sylvia recognized her oral communication skills during book tours for her first publication: "That [book tour] played to my strengths because it was me having to be articulate and present to rooms of thousands of people." Oral communication is an important factor in Sylvia's work as a school social worker, and she feels this strength allows her to communicate complex ideas to students and parents whom she works with, explaining, "I also feel like I have an uncanny ability to articulate things in a way that not everybody can."

Louisa has applied her oral communication skills at poetry readings and in her advocacy work and recognizes this as a strength in many situations, saying, "I have a knack for public speaking and know how to engage a room and facilitate conversations."

Interpersonal Skills

Interpersonal skills were identified by many of the participants, and these skills presented in interesting ways: some participants leveraged their people skills to get through difficult math classes, some used these skills because of a keen interest in people, and some described their empathy as a strength. James has found that he has strong people skills in the context of his work and is able to use those skills to communicate well with others in the workplace. Amelia's neuropsychological assessment revealed strengths in interpersonal skills, and she also has seen this as a strength in the workplace: "I'm good with people, I like to think. And so that's a strength that I've definitely honed over the years, especially working at the restaurant."

One interesting application of interpersonal skills was found in some participants' awareness of leveraging their people skills to get extra help in math or to hide their lack of understanding. Emma felt very strongly that her people skills allowed her to pass her math classes.

> It was being able to get the teacher to explain it again and again . . . and part of that was my people skills and being able to not annoy them or frustrate them too much, but also be able to get them to explain things in different ways to me.

In fact, she admitted that her use of those skills could sometimes be manipulative:

> I would go home and convince my foster parents [using my people skills] so they would end up doing my math homework, and then . . . coercing the teacher . . . not coercing, manipulating.

Sylvia also felt that using her people skills in math class could be viewed as manipulative:

> I kind of knew how to talk to my teachers in a way that they would give me the answer. Does that make sense? I was really good at reading my teachers and . . . I would ask questions, and then eventually they'd sort of just kind of give me the answer, you know? [That is] sort of how I would get through, sometimes.

Amelia believed building strong relationships with teachers through her people skills was a path to success: "One of the reasons I survived math was because I made sure the teachers liked me and knew that I was trying my best." She added that making sure that the teacher liked her, showing that she was working hard, and being helpful to the teacher ensured that they would be more lenient when she struggled. Amelia also leveraged her peer relationships in math class: "I'd tag along to my more math in-depth friends, the ones that knew what they were doing, [and ask], 'Can you help me?'" Using her people skills in group work also helped Amelia:

> [We] did group work together, kind of mooched off of other people's work. Because usually we would do it together and be like, 'Okay, that's the answer, I'll just write it down.' Sometimes we'd have group tests where the table would all do the test together. And so even though I usually . . . didn't know what was going on, I tried to figure stuff out . . . and then made sure everyone had copied it down so that we all had the same answer.

Like Amelia, Emma also used her skills in understanding and working with people to her advantage: "I specifically researched . . . 'How is this teacher going to test? How is he going to teach? . . . How can I make my way through this?' But it was really just study groups and sessions with people." Emma noted her interpersonal strengths in general saying, "I'm really good with people. I mean, I was in a master's program to be a therapist, but I've been known as the people whisperer for a lot of my life."

Many of the participants expressed having a keen interest in people. As noted in her profile, and very similar to the path that Emma was on at one time, Sylvia has a master's degree in social work and is employed as an elementary school social worker. She described her trajectory as:

> It just sort of naturally flowed that I kind of found myself doing social work. And when I really look back, that's kind of

what I'd been doing my whole life, in a way. All my jobs prior were pretty connected to working with people.

Emma noted that she has "an ability and a willingness to understand and to work to understand people," while Amelia shared, "I like asking people questions about themselves. . . . Or engaging with people in a way that it's not just a pass-by engage. . . . I like getting to know people."

Louisa also expressed a strong interest in psychology and shared that she often spends hours looking up information to learn more. When asked to elaborate on her interest in this area, Louisa shared:

> I think I've always been fascinated by what makes people tick. I've just always loved sitting back and watching people and sort of observing them. I take an interest in other people's lives. I've definitely struggled with mental health challenges myself, and other people in my life have, as well. And so, I've definitely exemplified the saying, "research is me search." Which is sort of an inside psychology joke. So yeah, but in general, I've just been really interested in people.

Empathy was a skill that many of the participants reflected on, with Sylvia noting that the challenges of her own experiences helped her to develop a strong sense of empathy.

> I have huge empathy, because [of] what I went through in school. I feel like I have a lot of extra empathy and understanding sometimes for what students are going through. . . . And so I'm able to connect with parents, like I'm able to explain for a kid, to a parent, what may be going on in a way that the parents are able to have empathy for their child.

Sylvia also noted:

> My learning disability and also having the book happen . . . I think, have helped me have a lot of empathy for kids who are non-traditional learners, . . . it doesn't really matter if they have

extreme strengths or low weaknesses. It's more just seeing all those bits and pieces of where kids are coming from.

Emma, as noted in her profile, has done advocacy work for trafficked women and children, which requires a great deal of empathy, and she has seen her sense of empathy as a way in which she's able to connect with people.

> I have an empathy and sensitivity and understanding [for] all sorts of people, of all different ages and experiences, or maybe [it's] not understanding right off the bat, but an ability and a willingness to understand and to work to understand people and to be with them where they're at.

Similarly, Louisa shares:

> I consider myself to be a rather empathetic and engaging person. I care deeply about other people and have a desire to help them. Because of my compassion, curiosity, and inquisitiveness, I'm good at asking people questions about how they're feeling.

In addition, Louisa is passionate about social justice and sees empathy as an important part of that work.

Creativity

Creativity showed up in many ways throughout the participants' interviews. They had similar experiences with music, theater, art in a variety of media, and creative thinking.

Many of the participants had hobbies and school experiences related to the performing arts and identified these hobbies and experiences as opportunities to tap into their strengths.

Playing music was one of Emma's hobbies. She is self-taught on guitar, ukulele, piano, and violin and also can play a little banjo and cello and stated:

> I taught myself all these instruments and can play them well. I cannot read music... I was in India, working with kids who

> had been trafficked, and there was a guitar lying around, and they needed someone to play guitar, so I just taught myself guitar, so that I could play music for the kids. But music . . . yeah, I can do this. I can pick up a guitar and figure out how to play it, . . . I love music and I love the instruments I play.

Amelia also has enjoyed music. She loves to sing, and she plays guitar and piano, on which she is largely self-taught. Amelia also participated in choirs in school: "And since I was very little, I started singing, and so they put me in choruses that I wanted to do or glee clubs." Amelia also had the opportunity to participate for a few years in high school in an Afro-Haitian music and dance ensemble, in which she excelled: "The second year I was the person that they would have show [others] how to do the movements, because I was doing well."

Just as with Amelia and Emma, music and dance have been an important part of Louisa's life, who stated:

> I don't play any instruments, but like I mentioned before, I do sing. I was in the school choir all throughout middle school and my freshman year of high school. I auditioned for regional music festivals in 8th grade, some of which I got into. . . . As far as dance is concerned, I danced in a local dance festival the summers before 8th and 9th grade. I was choreographed by a young dance major who had experience in choreographing people with cerebral palsy. Both dances were modern dance/contemporary ballet.

Three of the participants participated in musical theater. Louisa was involved in her school musicals between fifth and tenth grades, and Amelia says about her musical theater experience: "And then sophomore year, I auditioned for a student-run musical, *Carrie*, which I got the lead, [it] was my first audition." Sylvia participated in theater as a teenager: "Being involved with theater was really fun in high school. So that was something that I think also kind of played to my strengths."

Visual arts has played a role in the lives of many of the participants, both as a hobby and a career. Emma identified herself as a working artist and is currently writing and illustrating a children's book. She also enjoys art in her spare time: "I pack my bag with my sketchbook and everything and just kind of wander the woods, painting and imagining things." She was self-taught as an artist and has viewed art as an important part of her life:

> If you love something, you make time for it and you do it, and so, loving to draw and to paint, that's just something like, I'm going to do that every day, no matter what. Even if it means I'm going to bed later, that [art] is just a priority for me. But I've never taken any art classes or anything. It's all been kind of just setting aside time for myself and making that space for myself.

For Amelia, the joy of art has been in creating things with her hands, and her pursuits range from watercolor to crafts: "Everything there is creative I like to do, wax seals, I crochet, I make gloves, I knit, I make bookmarks. Basically, anything that I can do with my hands that's some form of art, I love doing."

At the time of her interview, Louisa's goal was to be able to support herself as a working artist with a focus on digital art. Toward that goal, she spoke about an upcoming exhibit of her work:

> Within the next month or so I'm going to be doing a local art show at the local library with a woman who happened to see my artwork on my social media and really liked it. And, she's an artist and she offered for us to collaborate on an art show together.

Art has always been important to Louisa and was reflected in her choice of extracurriculars in school:

> I also did photography and graphic design classes in high school. And I was nominated for a scholastic art award. My photograph didn't end up winning anything, but it did get sent up for submission. . . . I've always been a very creative person.

While Sylvia doesn't see herself as an artist, she has an appreciation for it, which she ties back to her experience in theater: "I've always loved art-related things. I was involved with the set crew and in charge of sort of managing that piece of it and that was fun for me."

Creativity was also evident in the ways in which the participants thought and their ability to creatively solve problems. Amelia, for example, has seen in herself an ability to take in important information and use that to her advantage to solve problems: "Noticing the details is something that I'm also good at, and seeing how things can work best."

In school, James feels he used his creative strengths to work around his challenges: "So I would say my strength in school was creativity and avoiding participating in programs that the school wanted me to participate in. Creativity and stubbornness." James's work as a software developer has required creative thinking and problem solving, which he identifies as strengths:

> Within pretty much any problem area that I've been able to engage in, I feel like I have an ability to do lateral thinking better than what I've seen in the workplace. So once I entered the workplace, I found that I was very, very strong in computers, but what I realized after a very little bit of time . . . was different about me, was that I could think laterally and put together connections. [That] has helped me to be the kind of person who can break down problems, which in software is critical. You actually have to break down the problems and think about them in very nonlinear ways.

When asked about her nonacademic strengths, Sylvia responded: "I think I'm pretty good with things like listening and creative problem solving." She described her ability to use this strength during a summer job:

> I worked at summer camp and I loved my . . . camp experience as a counselor. That was awesome. So you know that was fun and that played to my strengths, just because I got to do a lot of creative problem solving.

Creative thinking and problem solving have been also important skills in Sylvia's current job, which she recognizes as important strengths of hers.

> I guess what I call creativity is being able to just freely think and free associate . . . and looking at things from a very different perspective. When I'm trying to think about how I'm going to address an issue with a kid, I may not approach it in the most traditional manner. I might come up with something that's a little different, but it gets us to the same place than maybe a more traditional therapist might do. . . . You know, it's that sort of thing where you're kind of always thinking about intuitively, "What is it that I could do here? What could I use or manipulate to get to this issue for a kid or help them?"

Louisa articulated how creative strengths have benefitted her in her life by explaining:

> I think it's really given me an outlet for expression, and utilizes my skill of sort of outside-of-the-box thinking. I think I've always been really strong in thinking about new ideas and how to communicate in a way that when people see my work, they've been very intrigued at my sort of novel techniques, interesting ideas, etc.

As a person with physical disabilities, Louisa has seen problem solving and creative thinking in the ways that she has had to adapt to be able to do things that for others are easy: "I've also just been really proud of every milestone I've hit that seems so simple for other people, but it's not for me. I found other ways to get there on my own."

Opportunities to Develop Strengths and Interests

Opportunities to develop strengths varied widely between participants. For some, their strengths and talents were noticed by adults while they were still in school. For others, strengths weren't necessarily identified, but they had opportunities to engage in interests that were later identified as strength areas.

While in high school, James managed to get himself into an AP computer science class despite his academic challenges and identification as a special education student:

> Yeah, that was a freak thing. So sophomore year of high school while in special ed. and LD for everything else, I somehow got myself into the AP computer science class the first year they were running it for our high school, because I could do all the things that they needed to do.

James excelled in that class, and his high ability was noticed by the teacher, who allowed him to work ahead of the class at his own pace:

> I would just say that [during] the entire class I was mostly bored and reading chapters ahead in the book, because things were taking longer. I was off on my own the whole time and the teacher was completely fine with that. I just went and did my own things. . . . I did projects out of that book and enjoyed the book. And she was very happy with it, but she basically couldn't keep the whole class up to speed with the book. So, I pretty much ignored the lecture or just participated a little bit.

His teacher's recognition of his high potential in computer science led her to recommend him for an internship program:

> They had a program [where] the site scientists were needing people to do software development, and they were reaching out to schools to see if they could find somebody. Through that introduction, I ended up in that as a summer job, which I parlayed into [a paid job] . . . and worked there for four years doing software development for them.

James's experience with the internship-turned-job eventually led him to recognize his high ability in that area:

> I did not feel like I had any particular skills until I realized in my mid to late 20s that I had been working with people that [sic] had master's degrees in computer science from good universities. Then I did not feel at all that I was behind them.

When asked how that experience affected him, James reflected on the importance of that event in his professional life:

> Huge event for [me]. Basically, it allowed me to basically write my own story, . . . because once you get one thing and you get a success, that's how careers are, . . . you build the next, you build the next, you build the next, and then it snowballs from there.

Sylvia was fortunate that her gift for writing was recognized at a relatively young age, which allowed her to develop her talents with guidance from teachers. When asked about when she was first recognized as having strengths in writing, Sylvia remembers:

> I mean, [recognition of strength in writing] wasn't really until I started writing poetry. I did my first creative writing pieces in fifth grade. . . . I had a teacher finally say, "Don't worry about spelling and grammar, just look at this picture and write about it, I don't care about the other stuff right now." And that was the first aha moment for me, and then the teacher read it and went, "Oh, wow, this is great!" And I remember getting a lot of kudos for that and then producing more.

As she progressed as a young writer, Sylvia had a unique opportunity to write a book of poetry:

> So the first book . . . was kind of an odd project. So I had been struggling in school, and in eighth grade, I had a writing

> teacher who really was working with me . . . because I, at that point, had discovered creative writing, creative writing was great. I was struggling desperately in school with my learning disability. And so a friend of ours, who's a watercolor artist, gave me a rack of slides. . . . And I was writing poetry to those pictures. And then . . . my English teacher was helping me edit because that was one thing I didn't have experience with, editing my work.

As previously noted, Sylvia's first book was a success, which led to publication and speaking tours, giving her broader recognition of her talents beyond home and school. Thanks to her mother's advocacy, Sylvia had other opportunities to develop her writing as she grew up. One summer, she attended an out-of-state writing camp for gifted young writers, and, in high school one year, she was able to dual enroll and take a college-level poetry class.

Aside from her first book, one of the most important opportunities to develop strengths was presented to Sylvia through participation in Odyssey of the Mind, a competitive program for students to collaborate in teams on creative problem solving:

> It was like a game changer for me. It was the first time where I felt like I was with people who . . . were on the same page. [We were] just fully on the same page. I mean, I could get along with everybody else, . . . they were quirky and weird, different colored socks on different feet, you know what I mean? . . . And the sense of humor, we had the same sense of humor. . . . It felt like I finally found my people. That's how it felt. It really did. In fifth grade, that was huge. It was very cool, and I stayed involved with it for, I think, three to four years. Then the program faded out, unfortunately. But it was a big deal to be able to just freely let loose, because really, [the] sky was the limit in terms of what you could come up with. It was like, how magical is that?

Her Odyssey of the Mind experience not only helped Sylvia find and connect with like-minded peers but was also important in helping her understand herself and her unique strengths and challenges:

> I know I gained confidence. I think I gained a sense of just feeling connected to people, which hasn't always been easy for me. I think I felt like . . . it was an opportunity to get rewarded, I guess, for creative problem solving. . . . It was the first time I figured out different people have different strengths. There were two guys on the team who were just super into mechanical engineering. And they created their own . . . electromagnet thing that was going to pick up the things that we had, and so like everybody on the team had a different strength, and that was really a cool eye-opener for me.

Most of Louisa's opportunities to develop her strengths and interests came through classes and extracurricular activities at school. She took classes in photography and digital art and participated in choirs and musical theater. As noted earlier, Louisa recently developed a collaborative relationship with a fellow artist in her community. She hopes this collaboration and the subsequent art show will generate interest in her art so that she can eventually make a living with it. Louisa also attended disability leadership conferences in her youth, which she feels have given her skills for her advocacy work.

Emma's and Amelia's experiences are unique in that they were not aware of their giftedness until they received neuropsychological testing and were identified as twice exceptional at ages 26 and 18, respectively. Both participants were surprised by the gifted part of their identification and had not been recognized for any particular strengths while growing up. They cited no opportunities to develop strengths, as they had not yet been identified. In spite of this, Amelia had many opportunities to develop her strengths and interests through her participation in choirs, school musicals, and the Afro-Haitian dance ensemble.

Support Received During Schooling

Although some participants were not diagnosed with dyscalculia until later in their schooling or adulthood, all received support in some form. Some were put into special education math classes; some received tutoring from family, through school, or with a tutoring service; and for a couple of participants, creative scheduling allowed them to receive enough credits to graduate from high school and/or college.

Special Education

James remembered that his diagnosis of dyslexia, dysgraphia, and what at the time was referred to as "math dyslexia" resulted in being moved to a special education school:

> I was pulled out for testing early on in the third grade. I think it was actually . . . they moved me from the fourth grade to third grade. And in the testing, I was quickly identified . . . and then moved into a special education program at a different school.

In describing the special education school, James shared:

> They sent me to a different school that prided itself as basically being the magnet for learning disabilities. They had a [lower] teacher-to-student ratio, and we had basically a classroom and classroom assistant, and we had a smaller class size, and people spent a lot of time one-on-one. I have a lot of memories of flashcards . . . and people wanted to gamify the learning of the multiplication table. I felt like there [were] a lot of . . . young teachers who really felt like they were going to be the one that created the breakthrough that would help me learn the multiplication table. I'm sure I disappointed them through temper tantrums.

James was in special education from his diagnosis in third grade through high school, with only one experience in a regular education math class after his diagnosis:

> Actually, I think I attempted a mainstream geometry class because they were trying to mainstream kids out of special ed. I think I failed the geometry class and then I took a special ed. version of geometry and passed that.

When asked to reflect on his experiences in special education, James shared, "Math was just a shockingly bad experience." He felt that the attempts of the school to support him in math were a failure: "to say that I was not successful is . . . not an exaggeration. I was not successful in the special education classes at all." In elaborating on his attitudes about the support he received, James shared:

> I know it sucks to sound so bitter, . . . like every [intervention] that they did seemed to [have] failed. . . . It seems like if you would count up the number of hours that as a young child I spent trying to learn [math], the opportunity cost of that time has got to be huge, and it did not produce the result that all the people wanted, including [by] myself and my parents. Whatever other results could have been achieved in those times was lost, because it [was] a huge amount of wasted time. . . . I really just have such a negative view of the special ed. [of that] time. . . . I mean, it's not that they were bad people, it didn't work for me.

For Sylvia, math struggles had been a lifelong problem, and due to her mother's advocacy and insistence, she was finally evaluated, diagnosed, and placed in special education for math when she was in eighth grade:

> They finally realized I had a second-grade math level. I was trying to do eighth grade work, so they finally placed me in a special ed. math class . . . but essentially at that meeting, it was decided that because I was more than three years delayed, I could qualify for special ed. And so I officially became labeled with dyscalculia. I was officially placed in a special ed. math class.

When asked about in-school support prior to her diagnosis, Sylvia remembered:

> There might have been a couple of pull-outs that happened along the way, like resource room pull-out, you know, not special ed., but low groups. I was in a lot of low math groups going through school. They would group kids by ability, and I would get grouped in the lower group. I can't see that there was a lot of other support, because nobody wanted to recognize that I truly had this issue. So, they just treated me like I was your average student because nobody wanted to see it. I can't remember anything else happening until I got the special ed. support.

Any relief Sylvia felt about being moved to special education classes for math disappeared once she reached high school.

> And then high school, special ed. fell apart. By the time you get out of middle school, special ed. is not supported in the way that it is in elementary and middle schools. I would say for most schools in the country, that's kind of the way it works. By the time I was in high school, it was a joke. I mean, I would go to my special ed. math class, and there just wasn't anything really being offered . . . there were a lot of people who, I think, wanted to help, but then the help wasn't really available.

Although Louisa wasn't formally diagnosed with dyscalculia until the age of 21, her challenges in math were recognized very early in her schooling.

> I would say 6 years old [was when] they first started noticing it. I remember on my report card from first grade, it was repeatedly failing. It was repeatedly saying, [Louisa] is struggling in math and, but no one else really gave it much thought other than, "she's a bad math student. But, maybe she'll catch up." And then, as the year progressed, . . . I was sent out

> during math class sometimes. . . . And then [in] second grade, they started taking me out of math full time, and then [at] 8 years old, I was referred for formal testing. I started special education math when I was 7. It was apparent that there was a problem . . . when I was 8, but no one gave it a name until I was 21.

Louisa felt that her special education math classes were helpful, in part due to the extra assistance she received due to her cerebral palsy:

> I was in a special education math class that sort of remediated my curriculum down to four grade levels below what level my brain was. I was also given a one-on-one aide for my cerebral palsy since the age of five, and, . . . because I had the one-on-one aide, not only did they help me with, like, physical stuff, but conveniently they were also able to help me through math.

Louisa credited her special education services and aide with helping her pass her math classes saying, "I feel like if I wasn't given that, I would have metaphorically drowned. I feel like school would have been very, very difficult if I had not gotten those services. I probably would have failed math every year." Even though she had no formal diagnosis at the time, Louisa was fortunate that her math struggles were recognized by her school, and she was able to receive special education services for math from second grade through her third year of high school. Once she transferred to a therapeutic boarding school to repeat her junior year and complete her senior year, her math struggles were neither recognized nor supported.

Tutoring

Three of the participants spoke about receiving tutoring services, whether at school, with a tutoring service, or through family or friends. Perceptions were mixed with regard to the effectiveness of those experiences.

Sylvia remembers that her tutoring experiences were helpful, but not with math:

> I was doing Orton Gillingham tutoring at one point, outside of school, which did help me tremendously. My mom claims, I didn't know myself, I wasn't aware of myself well enough at that time, in terms of organization, but she claims that [it] made a huge difference for me with organization. It didn't fix the math issue, but it was insanely helpful for me with other pieces of my life.

Sylvia also remembered help from a specific teacher that was somewhat effective, though the teacher didn't seem to know how best to help her:

> My special ed. teacher in eighth grade . . . that woman was awesome, and she really worked hard. What she did was, I guess it's not rocket science, but she made me do sheet after sheet after sheet, just repetitive multiplication, or, not multiplication, [but doing] addition and subtraction sheets. I think that helped me cement those skills. She was constantly hitting me with those. So, she tried a lot of different techniques and [she] even kind of said to my parents, "There's just something here, there's a disconnect." I'm not sure even she had the answers of how to unlock or handle [the situation].

For Amelia, tutoring came mostly from family, though later from a service:

> There was tutoring at a certain point. My parents also didn't know what I was learning in math. They're like, "Ah, we can't help you anymore." . . . My older sisters helped me. I have two older sisters, so they helped me. Basically, wherever I got help, wherever I could get help, I would get it. Sometimes friends would help. But it was mostly tutoring. That [help] and in high school, I got tutoring help with math.

A major benefit of Amelia's tutoring experience through a neighbor's after-school program led to her eventual diagnosis. She described the experience as:

> She co-runs an after-school tutoring program, and she knows tons of stuff about ADD, ADHD, dyscalculia. So she also told my mom, "I think [Amelia] has dyscalculia," because I was tutored by some of her staff. She said, "Yeah, I think something's a little off.:

Emma had a set of foster parents she remembers as being patient and helpful with her math homework, saying, "[They] were really gracious and understanding, and . . . said, 'Okay, I'll sit with you and help you with this for hours at a time or whatever.'" Aside from that help, Emma has negative memories of tutoring and math support:

> Tutoring . . . was largely ineffective and I hated it. What works for me, and what's been most helpful for me even as an adult is thinking, "There's some part of me [that] kind of wants to be able to . . . , I don't know how to divide or multiply, and I want to be able to have those skills." Things like that. Part of what's most helpful for me is, even as an adult, to be able to manipulate objects and move things around and to build those skills. Tutoring was kind of just sitting with the math teacher, which I didn't like her anyway. Having to sit with her during study hall [with] me trying to get her to explain my math over and over and over again until I could understand it. . . . But mostly, it was like more math was assigned to me . . . [and] I get more worksheets and more math. [They said], "You're bad at this so here, do more of it. Have more of it to do at home and that'll help you."

Creative Scheduling

One of the more interesting types of support came in the form of creative scheduling, which essentially amounted to finding ways to work around required math credits for graduation. James and Sylvia both described this strategy as being responsible for their ability to graduate from high school and, for Sylvia, also from college.

When asked whether there were any supports that were helpful to him, James shared: "The topic of things that could help with math . . . the fact that maybe I was able to avoid those classes and still graduate high school was a help, that they had a program to waive it." However, James noted that his lack of exposure to regular education math was a significant roadblock to being able to be successful in college where math courses were a requirement.

For Sylvia, creative scheduling involved focusing on the courses that would meet requirements and doing alternative activities to get credits in high school. She explained:

> So a lot of creative scheduling happened for me, which means, my mom was handpicking. She'd go in and talk to the counselor. They would handpick my classes [such as] you can't take physics, but you can do X, so let's do that instead. There was a lot of trying to figure out how to help me graduate because in [my state], they had a ton of requirements for high school graduation, and I wasn't going to meet those in the traditional manner. So, they had to do a lot of fancy dancin' with the schedule.

Some of Sylvia's creative scheduling involved creating opportunities for her to receive high school credits by working with other teachers in their classrooms:

> At one point I was walking to an elementary school and I was doing kind of like an intern teaching thing with a second grade teacher. I'd go and help her out in her classroom. I mean, it was just really random stuff.

Sylvia was fortunate to attend a college that allowed enough flexibility for her to continue that strategy: "I always had to get cleared from the registrar, like, would these classes count. . . . So it was piecemealing my way through college, and it was literally just, again, creative scheduling." Sylvia added that through creative scheduling, she managed to avoid taking any regular education math classes after eighth grade and somehow avoided taking any math courses at all in college: "I don't know how that happened. . . . I literally don't know how that is possible. But the last math class I had, a gen. ed. math class, was eighth grade."

Emotional and Behavioral Responses

All of the participants had strong feelings about their experiences with dyscalculia and similar emotional and behavioral responses to the challenges they experienced in school. Many reported having worked very hard, feeling embarrassed, needing to hide their struggles, and feeling a great deal of frustration and anger.

Trying Hard

Many of the participants felt that although they were largely unsuccessful in their efforts, they tried very hard to learn math. James said he vacillated between caring and not caring but still put in a lot of work saying, "I'm still shocked to this day that I can't get it." He felt that in spite of his inconsistent attitude, he still worked hard: "People really put a lot of effort into trying to teach me the multiplication table, including myself."

Amelia stated that although she was struggling, it was important to try hard, and it was important that teachers recognized her efforts: "A lot of it was making sure that the teacher knew that I was doing my best and asking them for help and all that stuff." She put in a great deal of effort, but didn't see any progress as a result of her hard work: "I just . . . couldn't learn it in time, no matter how much I tried. It's not that I . . . wasn't trying, it's that I was trying it, I was trying my hardest, and it just wasn't good enough."

Sylvia put in a lot of time and effort, both at school and at home, but also saw little progress as a result: "There was my math teacher, my eighth grade math teacher, who said he'd never seen anybody work so hard and fail so much."

When Louisa was receiving support, she worked hard; however, once she transferred to the boarding school, she felt her attitude changed and she started putting in less effort:

> So what happened was I would go into math class raring to go, trying to get work done, and then getting really confused and asking for help and [the teachers] not knowing how to teach me math. When you have a person with a learning disability, people have to realize you need to teach this kid differently.

Faking It

Feeling embarrassed about their learning differences caused some participants to put effort into faking it as much as possible so that their peers wouldn't know they couldn't do math, both in school and in their adult lives.

James remembered feeling a need to hide his challenges when he started his internship: "It basically freed me from academics because they didn't know that I was a horrible student, yet I was performing really well there and I basically lived a dual life of hiding the fact that I [had learning differences]."

James continued his habit of hiding his learning differences into adulthood, though he feels more comfortable with himself now:

> I hid it for most of my career, including now. I'm sure that at work, people don't know. But I stopped caring about hiding it. . . . If you can hide some things, it's easier. So, it took me a long time to get comfortable with that.

Emma, who was honest about resorting to cheating to pass some high school and college math classes, felt that for most of her schooling she was pretending she understood and was hoping no one would notice: "I feel like I kind of just fudged my way through everything . . . everything was just faking and fudging and cheating in order to pass classes when it really mattered [in] high school and college." Even as an adult, Emma has found herself trying to hide her challenges: "I just have to fake and fudge, because there's no adult, there's nobody explaining to me. There's no other way to make sense of this."

Amelia recognized that at some point she began to try to fake her way through math class, although it was harder to do so when she was younger: "When I was younger, [it] was a lot harder, because I was less aware of how, I guess, different I was, or less used to pretending that I [understood] what people [were] talking about." She felt that she was able to hide in part due to her strengths masking her struggles: "Nobody really noticed anything because I was good at hiding it and [my strengths and weaknesses] kind of canceled each other out." Amelia believed that she developed skills using her strengths to hide her difficulties in math, saying she succeeded by:

> For lack of a better term, BS-ing. I've gotten really good at that . . . just kind of, saying the right words makes it seem like you know what you're talking about, even if maybe you don't. So, I've gotten good at making what I have work for me, and making the most of the little that I know or had.

Amelia was also able to hide due to the structure of some classes and a lack of oversight of her work:

> Luckily, I had the same teacher twice for two of my math classes. So that was helpful because he really knew me. I'm going to be honest here, for those two last math classes, he didn't really check the work, because sometimes I'd just scribble and stuff and pretend that I tried. If he had checked the work, I don't think I would have passed that class.

As a student, Sylvia worried that her classmates would find out about her struggles: "It made me feel like, 'Okay, are they going to find out that I can't do certain things?'" As a defense strategy, she tried to blend in and hide her challenges:

> [I was] pretending to look interested or look like I knew what was going on. Fearing to God that I would get called on to have to give an answer was . . . always like the biggest awfulness. There was a lot of just faking it till I made it through the hour of math. I mean, it was really painful.

Hiding was emotionally difficult, and like Amelia, Sylvia felt that she tapped into her strengths to hide her difficulties and blend in:

> I became an anxious, anxiety-ridden mess . . . full blown panic attacks, wasn't eating. I mean I was a disaster. I was a walking disaster. So I internalized all of that. I tried to hide. . . . I tried to pretend that I knew what was going on all the time. I mean, I used every strength I have to cover for what I couldn't do, as far as I could, but I always felt like I was a fake and an imposter because I knew there was the stuff I couldn't do.

During a college science course that included math, Sylvia once again used her strengths to try to hide the fact that she was struggling:

> I barely made it through my science class . . . because they had labs we had to do, and in the labs, they would expect us to chart things and do graphs and all this stuff, and I couldn't do it. So I would just sit there, and my lab partner . . . kind of had some strengths I didn't have and vice versa. But, had he [the instructor] come and questioned me directly to ask if I truly understood . . . you know? So there was a lot of just faking it. Pretending.

Sylvia viewed her ability to mask her difficulties as being a strength, both when she was a student and in her adult life:

> I would say that I am excellent at covering for my deficits, I'm really good at that. So I can come across as very articulate

and put together . . . and then, there's other things that aren't so put together.

As a student, Louisa did not want to hide her math struggles from her teachers but felt compelled to hide them from her classmates, in part because of the otherness she already felt having cerebral palsy:

> I wanted my teachers to know about it so that I could get the accommodations I needed. However, I did feel compelled to hide my dyscalculia from my peers in the mainstream classes I was in. I felt embarrassed by my dyscalculia and didn't want to feel like any more of a pariah than I already was—I already felt that way because of my CP. I couldn't hide my CP, so anything different about myself that I could hide, such as my dyscalculia, I did. I wanted to be as normal as possible; I already felt like a freak. As a result, I would change the subject when people would ask who my math teacher was.

As an adult, Louisa has struggled with deciding whether to hide or not:

> Now, as an adult, I do sometimes feel the need to hide my dyscalculia, but other times not. I often don't admit to people that I can't tell time or that I don't understand what they mean when they say "walk five feet this way" or give me rudimentary geographical directions that I don't understand. Sometimes I'll admit it, but it's embarrassing.

When asked to reflect on the ways that dyscalculia affects her adult life, Louisa shared how she felt about hiding her challenges:

> I would feel this impostor syndrome, like, "Oh my god, this person thinks I'm smart, but after [awhile], they're going to know that I'm not." And I'm [thinking], "Oh my god," so it's this anxiety about feeling like people are going to think I'm stupid.

Frustration and Stress

In addition to faking their understanding in math, participants often felt frustration as a result of not having their needs met.

James remembered what it felt like as a third grader struggling in school: "I was a disaster . . . I was a violent . . . frustrated young child that just did not fit in, fit in the world." As noted in his profile earlier, James was diagnosed not only with dyscalculia but also with dyslexia and dysgraphia. He felt that the way his school approached his dyslexia resulted in his healthy understanding of that learning difference, but the same was not true with regard to his understanding of dyscalculia:

> The issue of dyslexia was actually fairly well communicated to me, and I came to a reasonable understanding early on that not being able to spell, [it] didn't mean I was stupid. But early on in life, I really struggled with the idea that I wasn't stupid if I couldn't master the multiplication table. I thought there is no way that if I can't master the multiplication table, there's a level of stupid that I must be . . . as a young person, as a child, I would say that I waffled between just complete frustration with school all the time, going, "They're idiots" to "What's wrong with me? Why? . . . Am I not practicing enough or working enough?"

James felt a great deal of frustration with the education system as a whole and with what he saw as the skills being valued in school versus those that are useful in the world:

> I feel like [society is] rewarding exactly the wrong thing. If what we do is [take] little tiny children who are really really good at parroting back information, because they're good memorizers, and . . . [make them] report back information, [it's] a skill I wish I had. We tell them that they are smart and gifted people, so the kind of thinking that is valued is ignored and is [the kind of thinking] that I feel I was good at, and I am still frustrated by [that].

When reflecting on the impact of school on himself, James explained:

> I think that school . . . was the most damaging thing both to myself and my siblings. . . . I realized very early on that my difficulties were not associated with my intelligence, but I don't feel like the school ever realized those things.

Even now, James believes he has a better understanding of his strengths and his value, but he still struggles with his emotional response: "I just know that [schooling] is a huge thing and obviously continues to be a point of frustration."

School was also a frustrating and upsetting experience for Sylvia who said, "School was not an easy place for me to be, emotionally, physically. I mean, in so many ways, that was just such a tough, tough time." However, the increasing stress felt by Sylvia prompted her mother to insist on an evaluation from the school:

> I was starting to have panic attacks, not eating, and I was a total basket case. And my mom basically . . . put her foot down. She went to the director of special ed.'s office, [and she] said "I'm not leaving until you agree to do a grade level by grade level assessment of just math."

Amelia's memories of math reflected her frustration, anxiety, and confusion:

> I was coming home crying a lot, being stressed out about math . . . just intense stress from being absolutely clueless in math, even though we just learned it. And as soon as I finally kind of grasp[ed] the concept, they move[d] on to another unit, which was difficult.

She described her math experiences as a cycle of frustration:

> [The cycle was] can't figure it out, cry, still can't figure it out, cry, kind of figured it out, oh, the unit is changing, cry. So it was a lot of heartbreaking cycles there. I remember sometimes

taking tests in math and being on the verge of tears because I just didn't understand anything on the page.

Emma had clear memories of noticing that her classmates did not struggle in the ways that she struggled in math. Things seemed easy for them, and, more importantly, they were not worried about learning the skills and concepts. She didn't know she had a learning difference and couldn't explain why she was struggling, but she felt anxiety and pressure. She said, "I didn't know I had dyscalculia. There was no understanding of any learning disabilities there, but particularly dyscalculia." In her adult life, Emma still has felt anxiety around math, such as when she needs to measure while baking or cooking: "Those kinds of things are all very anxiety-inducing for me."

Much of Louisa's frustration lies in her awareness that she had potential, but her school was either unwilling or unable to accommodate her needs in a way that would have allowed her to work at a higher level:

> I really resent my school for what I'm about to tell you, which is the fact [that] they knew that I had issues with processing speed, which meant that it took a while for me to do my work. And the kids that had issues with that type of thing, like slow processing speed, were almost never in honors classes, even if they had the potential. I feel like the teachers didn't think to accommodate us. Accommodations would be like, less work, or a lot more time for homework or something. But they didn't do that. So I was thinking, I was like a really smart kid . . . with all these people that didn't have as much potential as me (sic). And my sister, and all these other kids that I felt like I could really relate to more, intellectually, were in different classes than me, and I just felt like I really didn't relate to anyone.

Louisa also expressed extreme frustration and anger about the fact that her boarding school did not recognize her math struggles and did not provide support: "[The boarding school] didn't think that I was having problems. They thought I was lazy, and I [thought] why did my other school catch this? . . . It made me very angry."

Some of the participants expressed frustration about the lack of awareness and understanding of dyscalculia. James compared understanding and acceptance of dyslexia with dyscalculia:

> I think dyscalculia did not and still does not have that level of acceptance that dyslexia has. I wouldn't have any problem if I explained to somebody in the real world that I am dyslexic. People would be like, oh, that's fine, I've heard of that. Dyscalculia, I feel like if I ran into somebody and just explained it to them, they'd be like, that makes no sense, and they would not believe . . . a lot of people would not believe that you could work as a software developer and have profoundly poor . . . math skills . . . [and] could actually do software that uses mathematical principles.

When asked if there was anything else she wanted to share about her experiences, Emma also compared the lack of awareness of dyscalculia to awareness of other learning differences:

> Just the lack of awareness and understanding. . . . Nobody knows what dyscalculia is. Nobody. There's just no awareness of it. Whereas, in general, people kind of have [an awareness of other learning differences], even people who don't have ADHD, or dyslexia, or whatever else. There's an understanding of what dyslexia is. I know this. But people don't know what dyscalculia is, let alone know it exists.

Sylvia connects the lack of awareness of dyscalculia to a lack of awareness of effective interventions and the difficulties that teachers face in trying to teach students with dyscalculia:

> You think "So, okay, you've got dyscalculia, so now what?" I mean, there really isn't a lot that I'm aware of, of different modes of intervening for kids that have that issue. So even in my own school, where I work, I have teachers come to

me and say, "Well, what did your teachers do for you?" [My response is] "not much, and we kind of just gave up."

Math Struggles

All participants shared that they had experienced considerable struggles with dyscalculia throughout their lives, both in school and in adulthood. Their struggles are mostly connected to numbers and math concepts and skills, but some of the participants also struggle in other areas that are not explicitly math related, such as with understanding time and scheduling.

School Experiences

When asked to describe their experiences as a math student, all participants have strong negative memories of being students in math classes.

Louisa's initial response to the question was laughter: "I'm sorry. I think I'm laughing because it's a really loaded question. [It's] nervous laughter. Math was really difficult and complicated." In elaborating on the experience, Louisa added:

> As far as ABCs and reading and stuff, we were doing that perfectly fine at the beginning. And then [with] math, it was like, the content was not only confusing, I was also really confused as to why it was confusing. I was so good at everything else and totally ahead of my class at everything else.... This doesn't make sense. It was like a weird cognitive dissonance. Wow, why do I feel smart and stupid at the same time? And it was just really frustrating. And, in fifth grade, for example, I had the reading skills of a 12-year-old, the writing skills of a 10-year-old, and the math skills of a 6-year-old. So it was like, what's going [on]? ... We were all just confused.

Like Louisa, Sylvia also remembered her school experience of math in a negative light:

> Oh, [it was] horrible. I remember wanting to do well. I thought I could do well. I never once thought that I couldn't

do it until I really couldn't, and even then I kept trying. It was tough. Math was hard. . . . I mean, there were other pieces to school that were challenging, too, because my brain just didn't do those things well, but the math thing was the main area that really was jacked up, for lack of a better phrase.

Amelia's memories of being a math student were directly to the point: "Math to me was just terrible." She also remembered feeling confused about her challenges: "It's always been difficult. I've always been the one that's just kind of clueless about what's going on in math class." Later, she added that she struggled to explain why math was so difficult for her:

I've always felt like small equations were difficult for me, or I just couldn't grasp concepts, and that was really difficult because I couldn't explain to people how I'm just not understanding what you're saying, and it's going in one ear and out the other.

Amelia's lack of understanding, coupled with her inability to articulate the problem, resulted in embarrassment:

I've always felt kind of embarrassed being in math class, because I was not understanding things, and I felt kind of stupid. I didn't know I had dyscalculia. I was, "Wow, I'm really bad at math, and everyone else is just okay and good at it."

Emma had vivid memories of noticing that her ability to comprehend certain things was very different from her peers, particularly with regard to time and the ability to subitize, although at the time she did not attribute those differences to math:

I noticed that there were, I wouldn't have called them math things, but I noticed that there [were ways] I was different [from] a lot of other people, [such as] with timing things. I don't have a very good sense of time. So I remember often [thinking] it's nine in the morning, but to me nine in the morning is the same as three in the afternoon. And so at school, I wouldn't necessarily say I didn't realize there was like a math or numbers component beyond [others' understanding and realizing that] everybody else is better than me, and they get this and I don't. It was more the things I noticed that really stood out to me, such as I don't have a sense of time. I don't know when three o'clock is going to come. Or, there's this, I think it's called subitizing, but [it's] the ability to look at a grouping of numbers and automatically [recognizing] this is five or whatever else. And so that for me where, again, I didn't connect it to math, [but it] made no sense to me. Now I can call it subitizing or whatever, but at the time, [my classmates could know] "Oh, there's five people here and so they need five plates for the dinner table" or whatever else, things like that. . . . Those are the two biggest things I remember pretty early on being [different from my] peers in understanding.

Emma also recognized a difference between her ability and her peers' ability when it came to more obviously math-related content: "So it's kind of like anything involving numbers was just kind of lumped away as, 'I'm bad at this, and all my peers and other people get it, and they understand it and I don't.'"

James remembered his early math experiences as being incredibly frustrating and his inability to understand why he couldn't master the skills or comprehend the content: "It just shocked me that I could not learn it." When James was still attending the school associated with the cult in which his family was living, James remembered being different from the other students in terms of academic ability:

[The school] actually had university-educated professors . . . a lot of the people there were high functioning academically. . . . So they had basically a Montessori-style school system that was a little bit more self-directed. I still have memories of it, but not great memories of it. And at that school, I was bizarro behind all the children in the measures of school. I had already known before we left the cult that I was sort of like a different child.

James's struggles in math, reading, and writing led to a diagnosis around third grade of dyslexia, dysgraphia, and what was called "math dyslexia." He remembered there was greater concern for his difficulties in reading than in math at the time but cited his inability to learn the multiplication tables in third grade as a factor in recognizing his math challenges: "I do know that the multiplication table was identified as [something] you're supposed to know."

Delayed Diagnosis

Louisa's math struggles were clear as soon as she began school, and she even received periodic academic assessments; however, despite the results showing a clear problem in math, no diagnosis was given. Louisa reported that the assessments showed "a severe discrepancy [with] above the average scores in verbal comprehension, [compared to] below average scores in working memory, processing speed, and math." She was perplexed that even though her math scores were significantly low, at less than the first percentile, the psychologist did not assign a formal diagnosis. Louisa speculated that the school psychologist likely did not believe there was a need for a diagnosis, but she disagrees:

> Maybe she felt like the descriptions [of behaviors] were enough to communicate the problem, and she felt like she didn't need to give it a name or something. But [it would] make it more simple, to say to somebody . . . like flat out, "Yes, I have a learning disability in math." But I felt like every time I said that to somebody, I was lying, or self-diagnosing, but . . . it was clear that they knew that I had dyscalculia.

Like Louisa, Sylvia's struggles in math were identified as early as kindergarten, and her testing also showed discrepancies between her challenges in math and high abilities in other areas. Sylvia's teachers interpreted the wide discrepancies in her early testing as those of an average student, and they dismissed the concerns of her parents:

> Kindergarten is when I think someone mentioned to my mom that she was noticing I was struggling. Then, first or second grade, they did a test, and I still have it somewhere, but there's the bars on the test [showing] the bars way up here for the language arts part, like way above average. Then there's the bars for the math, like way down here. They told my parents at the time, because I didn't fit anything with those scores, "Don't worry about it, she'll even out." That the two extremes will eventually "come to the middle" is literally . . . the quote that was stated to them.

When she was finally tested in eighth grade, Sylvia's school realized just how far behind she was in math: "I couldn't get past second grade math. Literally, they had me doing the workbooks. They had me start in kindergarten, first grade, second grade, and [continuing], from there, I couldn't go beyond that. "

Amelia also received testing that should have indicated a problem in math, but it was not diagnosed at that time:

> Yeah, [the problem] was suggested in eighth grade. When I got my first test done, it wasn't for everything, it was just specific, and my math grades were low, like really low, and they're like, "No, it's fine". . . but it was bad. For the neuropsych [assessment], I think I tested in the one percentile for math.

Amelia was diagnosed with dyscalculia during her senior year of high school when she had already completed the math requirements for graduation. She was not surprised by the diagnosis and lamented that she didn't receive the diagnosis and help much sooner. Emma believed that her delayed diagnosis was a direct result of having been in the foster care system for much of her childhood:

> With all the missed gaps and things from being in foster care, I feel like that helped things to kind of just be missed and

> explained away as another reason of, "Oh, well, you're in foster care and you've been bouncing around so your poor math skills make sense." Doesn't matter.... [It] was just kind of like, "You're bad at math, but who knows where you were [living] last month, so."

When asked if teachers ever noticed any red flags and brought that to the attention of her guardians, Emma remembered:

> Yeah, that happened frequently.... It was "You're failing math, you're not doing good in this." But then again, I think because of the foster care piece, switching schools and whatever else, and having different foster parents, it was never recognized or didn't carry on throughout my life.

Math as a Different Language

Emma and Louisa viewed math as being much like a foreign language that they are unable to learn. According to Louisa:

> I didn't understand why I didn't understand it. It was like learning a whole different language that everyone else seemed to get. And I didn't understand it, and I just felt like an idiot. Literally, I felt like an idiot.

Similarly, Emma expressed:

> The way I think of it and try and explain it to people is [that] numbers and math is like a whole different language to me, but not even a language that I can ever learn or know or understand or comprehend.

Math Struggles in Adult Life

All of the participants noticed challenges in their adult lives as a result of dyscalculia, though to varying degrees. For Amelia and Louisa, who are still living with their parents and are not yet fully independent, the challenges they experienced are minimal, but they both noted anxiety around their difficulties with life skills related to math. For Louisa, her challenges mostly related to an inability to read analog clocks, difficulty counting coins (both cognitively and physically), and understanding measurement and directions. When asked what presents challenges in her daily life, Amelia said: "I still have to count on my fingers. It's really difficult to do math in my head." She noted that she hasn't really had to do anything math-related since high school, though her job requires counting tips on occasion, and she worries about the accuracy of her counting: "I do have to sometimes count tips at work, and I'm like, quadruple check. And I even ask somebody else, even if it's like counting a few dollars, just because I'm, like, what if I'm getting it wrong." In general, Amelia noted that she struggles with time, counting, and calculations:

> [Counting tips] . . . also reading analog clocks. I have to count and add up everything. Reading big numbers, like millions, I've just never really done [those things], and so I don't really know how to do it. . . . Simple addition, sometimes I try to do it and all I'm hearing is words. And then in my head, my head is just not processing, so I have to close my eyes and really, really think about, like, the simplest subtraction and addition and multiplication.

James indicated that he struggles with calculations and still uses his fingers to calculate even single-digit problems: "Who the hell subtracts those two numbers and counts on their fingers, and I do, for even single-digit numbers, I count on my fingers all the damn time." He also notes that he has trouble with budgeting and time, particularly with scheduling:

> I miss meetings on a regular basis, maybe a little bit more than [other] people. You know, that's how you know that a meeting's important or not important, if you missed it and you get away with it, it wasn't an important meeting.

However, James doesn't believe these problems were significant in his daily life: "This is gonna be a huge problem, I thought. But it never was a problem. Like zero problems in my life have ever been related to math, you know?" James recognized that one impact on his adult life is centered around confidence issues, but it has served to guide him toward strategies to overcome his challenges: "Confidence problems around math created an issue I would say that I've [had] . . . the knowledge that I'm bad at it impacted me by basically guiding me towards coping strategies."

Sylvia and Emma noticed a much larger impact of dyscalculia on their daily lives. Sylvia noticed that she struggles with budgeting, with understanding elapsed time and scheduling, and with tasks that involve measurement. With regard to scheduling, Sylvia noted: "I can't always plan, like, timing things out is challenging, sometimes planning things out, planning out my day to know how much time I have to actually get something done." Difficulties understanding measurement has been a problem for Sylvia in multiple contexts:

> I mismeasure. I forget ingredients sometimes. I mismeasure, [and] that's a big thing. When I'm tired, too, oh my god, that's when mistakes really get intense. So yeah, I will mismeasure things. Cooking is an issue, quantity and volume, I'm not always good at judging like, how much do I need to actually make this work? I hate ordering things online because of sizes. I have to have a measuring tape by me all the time, like if I'm ordering rugs, or I'm ordering [something], I mean, I know that's probably [an issue for] most people, but when I read what a size is online, it means nothing to me. Whereas to someone else it'll be, "Oh, that's really tiny," you know? I'm like, "Is it tiny or is it big?" I don't know. I have no idea. So, sizing things, ordering things, trying to figure out what will fit, what won't? That is a big problem. Spatial stuff in terms of size, measuring is difficult. . . . I hate measuring things. Measuring things is a problem and reading the measuring tape [is] another issue.

> Sometimes just reading the measuring tape [is] knowing "Is that right or not right?"

Sylvia explained that there are often unexpected situations in which dyscalculia is a problem:

> You may not have the skills to meet that need, right? So, like airports are a great example. You get in the airport, and I may not know if the gate I need to get to falls within the [range of] numbers that they put on the sign, to gates 80 through 100. Well, I don't know if gate 79 fits in that window or not. So it's all these weird things that pop up in your daily life [which] are challenging.

Emma related daily challenges in things like calculating tips: "Yeah, there's been instances where I've tipped like, more than the bill, or things like that." Like Sylvia, she also has noticed difficulties with measurement and scheduling:

> So when I got married, I didn't own any measuring cups or spoons. And my husband was "That's weird, why don't you have measuring cups or spoons?" Well, it's because the fractions and everything, and the timing of baking or cooking. Baking, cooking, those kinds of things, are all very anxiety inducing for me.

In elaborating on how time and scheduling can be a problem, Emma said "I've done things where I'll schedule a dentist appointment and acupuncture with, like, 15 minutes in between, which . . . [means] there's not even enough time for the appointment, let alone to get from one place to the next."

Similar to Sylvia's challenges in locating a gate in an airport, Emma has struggled to locate the posted speed limit on her speedometer when she's driving:

> And then there's the whole, whatever it's called, that thing with the numbers that's like . . . speedometer, maybe it's a

speedometer. So, by the time I look at it . . . it doesn't have every single number up to 100. So that's a problem. And then to gauge passing speed limit signs, that sign that says 50, I can't find . . . the 50 on the speedometer.

Other issues associated with driving stemmed from Emma's difficulties with direction: "Driving is like a real difficulty for me with, like, left and right, and then even the GPS is largely unhelpful, [such as] on Apple, on maps, or whatever. Doesn't really work for me."

Like Sylvia, Emma also has taken a holistic view of the impact of dyscalculia on her daily life:

> [Even] my husband [will say], "Oh, well, why does it matter? You're an adult now," [but] the ways dyscalculia impacts me really now as an adult aren't necessarily solvable or. . . . It's more just like how it impacts my daily life, which isn't necessarily math related. . . . It's more the things that aren't necessarily related to math that impacted me in my adult life.

Sylvia also talked about the impact of her math struggles on her relationships, both in childhood and as an adult. With peer relationships growing up, she says,

> It was exhausting. It was, I think it hugely impacted me socially. I mean, I already struggled socially because I was never like your super outgoing kid, I was more of an introvert to begin with, but then the math piece again, it made me feel like, even with peers, like okay, are they going to find out that I can't do certain things?

Her math difficulties also impacted her relationship with her parents, as well as the shaping of her identity:

> And then there's another layer people don't always talk about, which is the whole parent relationship, right? Because when you do have significant deficits, you sort of need your parents, you need someone to help you with things,

and beyond what's developmentally typically considered normal. So that's a whole other level that not everybody thinks about. And you have to deal with that with your identity going forward into adulthood. And that was the biggest thing for me was [the] identity stuff. In college, that's when the identity stuff was huge, because I thought, well, I could go away to college. I went off to school . . . far, far away from [home], and I thought, "I'll go to school and everything will be great." You know, I'm leaving, I'm leaving my old world behind. So then that means I'll be fine. And what a silly thing, right? Because you go wherever you go.

Sylvia also saw dyscalculia as having a significant impact on her dating life:

It does impact your relationships, because . . . all of our weaknesses impact relationships, but if you are in a significant relationship with somebody, they're impacted, too, by your deficit, right? So that's a whole other piece. I mean, you're adding this level of responsibility to someone's plate . . . I know in my last relationship . . . he was a math professor, actually, so that worked out well. But, you know, when you really look back, it's kind of like, . . . that's a lot to take on for a significant other, right? And we all take it on for each other in those relationships, but, I always think about as an adult . . . that's probably one of the bigger areas that it impacts is your relationships, because if that person doesn't fully understand or fully get or is empathetic to [your challenges] it can create conflict, it can create a lot of issues, because they don't get it or understand.

Strategies for Navigating Adult Challenges

All of the participants have developed a wide range of strategies to enable them to overcome the challenges presented by dyscalculia in their adult lives.

James, who works in a field that requires some amount of math, said, "So the coping strategies for math was (sic) basically, always have a computer . . . which was great because I entered into a field [of] software development." In addressing how he does the math necessary for his work, James offered: "Math is something that's involved in software development. We do math, but arithmetic operations are not done . . . so I just avoid it . . . If I have to do math, I've got software to do math." Avoidance was a strategy that James found useful, both in his work and in daily life: "And never be the guy that, like, calculates things in your head, because you know you're gonna be wrong. Like, I can't calculate tips." Avoidance also came into play in James's strategy for budgeting and balancing his checkbook: "It's easier to balance my checkbook if I just never ever balance my checkbook. And then I just have a rule that says I keep $10,000 in the bank account." Using a calculator helps James whenever he needs to calculate something, a strategy he joked that teachers didn't anticipate when he was younger: "Oh, my teacher said that you won't always have a calculator, right? And of course, nowadays, [you] always have a calculator around you."

Amelia's strategies revolved around her needs in the restaurant where she works. Aside from checking her calculations multiple times and asking a coworker to verify her result, Amelia relied on technology to do math for her:

> Luckily, we don't take cash at work, we only do cards, everything's online. If it were cash, that would be a whole other story. Adding all that up would be terrifying. So luckily, that's good. And splitting a check, there's already a button that's in there. So we just have to press that and not actually split it ourselves. So really, there's not much math I have to do on a daily basis, which is really lucky for me.

Like Amelia, Louisa hasn't identified many challenges in her daily life, and her strategies for addressing them have also relied on technology:

> Luckily, clocks are for the majority digital, but some clocks are not. And I have to ask, "What time is it?" And, they'll

say, "There's a clock there," and I'm too embarrassed to tell anyone that I can't [read it] . . . [and] I usually use my debit card at a register.

For Louisa, the most important strategies she cultivated was knowing when to ask for help and being patient with herself:

> I've learned to give myself permission to ask for help. Like, "Hey, I actually can't do this, so I don't know what you're talking about," and I just have to be [thinking] "It's okay" or "you can wait like two minutes, check your phone, and there's a digital clock on there," or "you can use a calculator," [and] thank goodness for your debit card. . . . So there's [also] things that I'm just [thinking], "You don't have to do everything that a non-disabled person can do." Something that all of my life, since preschool, with my CP and later my dyscalculia, and other stuff, I've had to realize, "It's okay if you can't do this. It's okay if you need to wait to use a calculator or until you can get access to a digital clock, or you don't want to waste time making your fingers and your brain figure out how to manipulate coins."

Most of Sylvia's strategies for coping with challenges were related to her difficulties with time and scheduling:

> I've had to develop an intuitive sense of time, because clock time doesn't always register for me in the same way. So, I'm always having to [think] After you do enough cleaning of your house, you kind of know about how long that takes, but it's sort of this intuitive thing. I never fully know if I have enough time to do things. That's always an issue. But I've gotten better, I really have, with practice over time as an adult. Routines are super important for me. So, routines keep me grounded and keep me in place, and being routinized is a big part of survival when you have a deficit like that, because it's predictable. Unpredictability is like the nemesis [for] people who struggle.

An important strategy for Sylvia has been relying on her mother for things she cannot do herself:

> I'm still so dependent on my mom for help with my financial stuff. I need help with just budgeting, finances, [and] managing. A lot of those pieces [make me] still very dependent. So I'm dependent on her for that help. Lord help my brother when she kicks it, because, you know, I guess, I don't know.

Sylvia also relies on coworkers to make sure she doesn't have errors in her scheduling: "I have to talk out loud sometimes [about] my schedule to make sure it'll all work and have someone else tell me, 'Yes, that will work.'" Sylvia felt that awareness of anxiety and taking care of her mental health were among her most important strategies:

> I've learned as an adult that I have to be very aware of my stress levels and the impacts that anxiety has for me. I know that I've taken on too much and I'm trying to do too much when I start to have that mental health piece of it and anxiety creeps back in. I have to be very aware of that in my adult life. It's kind of like alcoholism, you're always recovering from anxiety. You're always having to be aware of it, and you always have to kind of watch, and do self-care around it, so I can't take on as much as I think other adults can. I don't know how [other people] juggle all of it. They have like three kids and a dog and a house and a husband, and I don't know how many other things [are] going on in their lives. I don't think I could cope. I can't cope like everybody else with all of that. So, my life's a little more limited, I think, from that perspective.

In spite of her challenges, Sylvia believed that as an adult, she has become much more comfortable acknowledging her limitations and asking for help: "You know, luckily I'm an adult now and I know that I would feel okay asking someone [for help], but when I was younger, I'd be mortified."

Some of Emma's strategies for dealing with mathematical challenges were quite typical, such as using calculators and debit cards: "I mean, calculators are just [a] gift from God. I use a calculator for most everything." She adds: "If I'm at the grocery store, I use a credit or debit card to pay. . . . But really, it's just a calculator that solves most things that are explicitly related to math." With regard to her difficulties with scheduling, Emma needed to be very intentional about her calendar and accept that she'll sometimes get it wrong and need to cancel or reschedule appointments. In cooking and baking, Emma struggled with measurement, understanding oven temperatures, and following the length of time indicated in a recipe, but she has developed strategies that work for her:

> I bake and cook, [but] I never measure anything. I use my Time Timer for if I need a specific time in the oven. But, I'll have to be really careful to make sure that if the oven is supposed to be at 725 or whatever, that I actually [set it at the] actual baking [temperature]. I have to be really careful that I actually look at the cookbook or whatever and put it there with the actual baking time. I use the Time Timer a lot for that. I've eliminated the use of measuring cups or spoons because they don't work for me. So I kind of cook and bake by sight and taste and with my own measurements, using my hands or just a regular spoon.

For driving, Emma developed creative strategies to address her difficulties with understanding speed limits and following directions.

> I have put additional little stickers for more numbers [than what is] on my speedometer, so that I can more quickly match the numbers [with the posted speed limits]. Or I'll find a car to drive behind that, hopefully, is going the speed limit. Things like that. I'm very directionally challenged, but for me that means instead of relying on left, right, north, south, east, west, I kind of [rely on] "Oh, the yellow house over there, turn towards the yellow house."

For addressing her difficulties with elapsed time, Emma tapped into her visual and auditory strengths:

> I have music playlists for certain amounts of time. I'm very visual and auditory, so I have my Time Timer that will show me, like, 30 minutes till I need to leave for this place or whatever. And then I also have playlists of standard lengths of time that I'll play, if it's something more like that.

Like Sylvia, Emma also relied on others for tasks she cannot do herself: "My husband takes care of budgeting and those kinds of things to do with numbers."

Summary

All participants provided important insights into their lived experiences as students growing up in educational systems that were ill-equipped to meet their needs and as adults navigating the challenges of twice exceptionality. The participants were unique in many ways, including their diagnoses, geographic regions, careers, and age at diagnosis. However, many insights, perspectives, and experiences were common among them. All participants had difficult experiences in school, have struggled to reconcile their high abilities with their extreme challenges in building healthy self-concepts, and have experienced a significant level of frustration and anxiety as a result of dyscalculia and the ways in which their needs were not met as students. Additionally, there were common strengths and interests among the participants, particularly with regard to language skills, interpersonal skills, and creativity.

5
Lessons Learned

What can we learn from the lived experiences of the individuals whose stories are shared here? The themes that lend themselves the most to furthering understanding of unique lives of gifted adults with dyscalculia include strengths potentially associated with dyscalculia, the importance of creating opportunities to develop strengths, emotional and behavioral responses to struggles with math and math-adjacent skills and content, and navigating the adult challenges presented by living with dyscalculia. This chapter discusses these conclusions in the context of the established research and the theoretical framework.

Positive Psychology

Positive psychology, the theoretical framework for this study, assumes a holistic view of the individual, with a focus on recognizing and understanding strengths, rather than solely focusing on deficits. Much of the research on dyscalculia is deficit based; however, positive psychology presents a research-supported perspective that individuals can better reach their potential when attention is given to recognizing and developing strengths (Seligman & Csikszentmihalyi, 2000). When balanced attention is given to both strengths and deficits, students are more likely to be successful (Baum et al., 1997; Olenchak, 1995). Furthermore,

DOI: 10.4324/9781003527800-5

when there is a balanced approach, strengths can be leveraged to address challenges (Peterson, 2009).

The participants in this study were all identified as twice exceptional. Many of the experiences they related pointed to years of frustration and stress in school and in life due to their inability to learn math in the ways it was taught to them, embarrassment over their learning differences, and confusion about their own intelligence and potential. For those participants whose strengths were identified and nurtured, there was clear evidence that they were better able to reach their potential. In addition, there was evidence that they were able to leverage strengths, such as interpersonal skills, to address the challenges they faced.

Lesson 1: Gifted Individuals With Dyscalculia Have Unique Strengths

The first theme that emerged from the data was identification of potential strengths of gifted individuals with dyscalculia. While conclusions about the strengths of dyscalculia are difficult to generalize based on a handful of individuals, naturalistic generalizations can be made from the experiences presented in the case studies. Additionally, the common strengths identified across cases confirms observations made by psychologist Dr. Stephen Chou from his work with 2e individuals with dyscalculia at the Summit Center in California and in his private practice. Dr. Chou explained that in his experience, gifted individuals with dyscalculia tend to show strengths in multiple areas, including innovation, intuition, social-emotional skills, interpersonal relationships, and verbal skills. His belief is that because these individuals are unable to use linear, sequential thinking, they use other parts of their brains that support these strengths (personal communication, January 19, 2022).

The participants demonstrated a pattern of strengths in a number of areas, including language skills, specifically writing and communication; interpersonal skills, including empathy and an ability to leverage these skills in challenging situations;

and creativity, including an interest in pursuits involving performing and visual arts, as well as creative thinking and problem solving.

Language Arts and Writing

All participants had evidence of strengths in writing, with four of the five identifying themselves as writers. Sylvia published two books, James and Emma were working on books, and Louisa received recognition of her writing ability through awards and a published poem. Most of the participants recognized their strengths in language and writing from an early age. Amelia did not; however, her neuropsychological evaluation provided ample evidence for superior to very superior ability in that area.

Interpersonal Skills

All of the participants identified people skills in one or more contexts. The evidence for interpersonal skills presented in surprising ways that also supported an argument for problem-solving strengths, with Sylvia, Emma, and Amelia explaining how they leveraged this skill to get through their math classes. Their strategies included (1) developing positive relationships with teachers so that they would be more likely to provide needed support, (2) researching the teaching styles of teachers to select professors who were a better fit, (3) relying heavily on group work, and (4) manipulating interactions to elicit answers from teachers and parents.

Creativity

Creativity was a common theme among participants. Four of the participants pointed to a love of art and rich and meaningful experiences with performing arts and/or visual arts in school and in their adult lives. Creativity was evident among the participants in other ways as well, specifically in the ways they think and their problem-solving ability. Additionally, creative problem solving was evident in the ways in which some participants navigated challenges in their adult lives, such as in the ways that Emma created work-arounds for her challenges with time management by creating music playlists or supplemented her car speedometer with additional numbers on stickers to support her difficulties with driving the speed limit.

There is considerable research that provides evidence of the identification of strengths associated with other learning differences. For example, Eide and Eide (2012) have identified dyslexic strengths including material, interconnected, narrative, and dynamic reasoning, which they term MIND strengths. Those with dyslexia have also been identified as having strengths in "big picture" thinking (Schneps, 2014), as well as visual-spatial strengths (Armstrong, 2010; Rappolt-Schlichtmann et al., 2018). Individuals with attention deficit hyperactivity disorder (ADHD) are recognized for their abilities in logical reasoning, emotional intelligence, and creativity (Climie, 2015). They are also known to have strengths in divergent thinking and an ability to get into a "flow" state (Armstrong, 2010). Autistic individuals are recognized as being able to be adept at detail-oriented and systematic thinking (Wright, 2013). Evidence of strengths of dyscalculia, however, is difficult to find in the literature. Only one study was found that successfully reframed dyscalculia as a cognitive difference rather than a deficit, and the authors discussed dyscalculia in a positive, strength-based light (Lewis & Lynn, 2018).

Lesson 2: Finding Opportunities to Develop Strengths Is Essential

The second lesson to emerge was related to the value of participants' opportunities to develop their strengths and talents. Opportunities varied widely among participants and seemed largely connected to whether and when their strengths were identified. Identification of strengths in twice-exceptional students is essential for healthy development of motivation, self-efficacy, and self-esteem, and this plays an important role in an individual's growth and future success (Baum et al., 2017). In fact, for those participants whose strengths in this study were identified by adults when they were younger, they recognized gifts and talents in themselves and saw themselves as gifted.

Emma and Amelia, for example, whose giftedness was not recognized until ages 26 and 18, respectively, had a harder time than the other participants viewing themselves as gifted or having high potential. James found the word "gifted" to be problematic, but his recognition as talented with computers in high school created opportunities for him to develop that strength, and he readily acknowledged his talents. Sylvia had the most opportunities from a young age. Her participation in Odyssey of the Mind helped her to connect with like-minded peers, and she saw herself as a capable, creative problem solver. Her recognition by teachers for her gift in writing led to an incredible opportunity to become a published author while still very young.

Researchers discuss the importance of identifying and cultivating strengths in 2e children, which can lead to increased academic achievement and a positive self-concept (Baum et al., 1995; Olenchak, 2009; Reis et al., 2014). A focus on strengths can serve to develop the capabilities of individuals who are more engaged and more successful (Reis et al., 2014). Additionally, recognizing the strengths of twice-exceptional individuals contributes to stronger social relationships; an improved ability to deal with social, emotional, and cognitive challenges; opportunities to form professional relationships with adults through mentoring; and the development of expertise in talent areas (Baum et al., 2014).

Lesson 3: These Struggles Impact Mental Health and Self-Concept

A third lesson to emerge from the findings was related to the emotional and behavioral responses of the participants to their experiences in math, which had an impact on their mental health and played a role in shaping their sense of self. There were common experiences of feeling embarrassed and the need to hide their learning differences from peers and feeling significant levels of frustration, stress, and anger from not having their needs met. Additionally, the participants felt there is not enough awareness and understanding of dyscalculia.

Embarrassment, Hiding, and Frustration

Even as adults, there were common experiences of still feeling embarrassment over their inability to do math or other tasks affected by dyscalculia, and they struggled with the urge to try to hide their challenges. Louisa spoke about being embarrassed when asked the time and her inability to follow simple geographical directions. Emma indicated she still feels compelled to "fake and fudge" and laments that, as an adult, there is no other adult to help her understand. Sylvia viewed her ability to hide her struggles as a strength that she leveraged in school and in adulthood.

Frustration and stress from not having their needs met was an ever-present experience for the participants. James shared that he responded to his frustration with a lot of anger and viewed his educational experience as the "most damaging thing" in his life. He indicated that he still feels a great deal of resentment toward the education system. Sylvia's stress increased to the point of panic attacks. Amelia's memories of school included a lot of crying from frustration and stress. Emma felt strong anxiety and pressure, which she still experiences as an adult when faced with tasks that are difficult for her due to dyscalculia. For Louisa, her frustration stemmed in part from not having adequate instruction and being called lazy at her boarding school. She was also frustrated because of her awareness that she had high potential but the schools she attended did not recognize her strengths or provide opportunities for her to grow.

For all participants, there was a clear impact from their frustration and stress on their mental health and the shaping of their sense of self. James believed that the education system harmed him, and he shared that he acted out violently as a child. Though he recognized his strengths now, he still struggles to understand his dyscalculia and thought that it "makes no sense" that he can't do certain things. In spite of a neuropsychological evaluation identifying Emma as twice exceptional, she struggled to identify as a gifted person. She is curious about what opportunities she may have missed out on from her delayed identification as gifted and doesn't know how to reconcile her giftedness with her learning difference. Like Emma, Amelia's identification as twice exceptional was a surprise, and even today she has difficulty accepting herself as gifted. She felt cheated by an education system that didn't recognize who she was or help her to grow. Like Emma, Sylvia struggled to reconcile her giftedness with her dyscalculia and says she has never felt "completely blended." Louisa described herself as having a confused sense of self and struggled to understand how she can be so smart and still not do certain things.

Existing research provides support for the importance of identifying twice-exceptional students and providing support from a strength-based, talent-focused perspective. A strength-based lens has been shown to increase academic achievement, as well as to support development of a positive self-concept (Baum et al., 1995; Olenchak, 2009; Reis et al., 2014). A focus on twice-exceptional students' strengths also supports development of their gifted characteristics, as well as higher engagement and a higher chance of success (Reis et al., 2014). In addition, research demonstrates that there are many benefits of a strength-based, talent-focused approach to education, including improved social relationships; stronger resilience in dealing with social, emotional, and cognitive challenges; and a higher chance of developing expertise in strength areas (Baum et al., 2014).

While the literature regarding a strength-based lens of dyscalculia is sparse, there is some evidence of the benefits of this approach for this learning difference. Intervention for students with math learning differences that focuses on strengths provides better support for deficits and builds motivation, while emphasis on deficits leads to decreased motivation and increased risk of failure (Karagiannakis et al., 2014). Also, a focus on strengths, through the lens of multiple intelligences theory, demonstrates higher math achievement for students with dyscalculia (Al-Zoubi & Al-Adawi, 2019).

Ineffective Interventions

All participants experienced inadequate, ineffective interventions in school and felt frustrated by their schools' inability to meet their needs or recognize their strengths. In addition, many suffered from the effects of a delayed diagnosis. With the exception of Louisa, who felt that one-on-one assistance from her aide was helpful, the participants all expressed frustration that their schools and teachers were unable to provide the kind of support that would help them to be successful in math. James and Emma spoke about feelings of confusion over why they couldn't learn math in the ways that their peers seemed able to do. Although Louisa felt that she had adequate support from her aide in her early schooling, her challenges in math at her boarding school were attributed to laziness and she was told to work harder. Emma remembered that her teachers tried to help her by giving her more math work to do. Sylvia recalled her tutoring experiences as being helpful for organizational skills but not for math. In her current job as school social worker, Sylvia said she sometimes has colleagues ask for suggestions on how to help students struggling with math, and she has nothing to offer from her own experiences as a student. When asked what her teachers did to help her, all she can say is "not much."

Not only did the participants experience delays in being diagnosed with dyscalculia, they also either experienced delays in identification as gifted or, in some cases, were never formally identified as such. In some cases, their strengths were not obvious to teachers, and in others, the educators at their schools were not trained to interpret the discrepancies they demonstrated. Authors discuss the importance of training to be able to identify twice-exceptional students and to make appropriate diagnoses (Mundt, 2014; Ottone-Cross et al., 2016; Cain et al., 2019). Studies show that while there is some awareness of 2e, not all educators and professionals are well-trained in understanding this population, with gifted specialists typically displaying deeper knowledge than special education teachers and even psychologists (Foley-Nicpon et al., 2013). Cain et al. (2019), in speaking specifically about under-identification of gifted individuals with autism, place blame squarely on a lack of training.

Delayed Diagnosis

For many students with dyscalculia, diagnosis occurs when problems arise around second or third grade; however, for many gifted students, problems may not be evident until at least middle school (Knop & Chou, 2020). James was diagnosed with dyscalculia, dyslexia, and dysgraphia around third grade, but the others experienced significant delays in their diagnosis. Louisa and Sylvia were showing signs of struggle as early as kindergarten but were not diagnosed until age 21 and eighth grade, respectively. Amelia was diagnosed in her senior year of high school, and Emma at the age of 26. These four participants felt frustration that they were demonstrating a clear need for intervention but for the most part were not receiving it. Louisa felt validated when she finally received her diagnosis, but she felt the damage had already been done, especially when attending the boarding school that labeled her as lazy and refused to provide support. Amelia expressed that an earlier diagnosis "would have been really helpful." Emma's response to discovering the existence of a math learning difference just prior to her eventual diagnosis at age 26 was emotional. She immediately recognized herself in the description, cried, and said, "This is me."

There were a variety of reasons for each participant's delayed diagnosis, from chalking up problems with math to an unstable home life in the foster care system, to misinterpretation of discrepancies in testing, to the possibility that their strengths masked their challenges to some extent. There is often confusion surrounding students with wide discrepancies between their high abilities and deficits due to a lack of understanding of twice-exceptional students (Gilger et al., 2008). Many of the participants felt that their strengths helped mask their challenges, at least to a point. Knop and Chou (2020) make reference to the possibility of "stealth dyscalculia." They believe that it is possible that a diagnosis of dyscalculia may be delayed in gifted students due to their giftedness or access to effective accommodations (Knop & Chou, 2020). In addition, for twice-exceptional students in general, it is common for their strengths to mask their deficits and for their deficits to mask their strengths (Reis et al., 2014).

Lack of Awareness

James, Sylvia, and Emma also shared that part of their frustration is rooted in a lack of awareness and understanding of dyscalculia. James compared his experiences with dyslexia and dyscalculia.

He felt that most people showed a level of understanding and acceptance of his dyslexia but believed that, for most people, dyscalculia "makes no sense." Emma also lamented that there is widespread understanding and growing acceptance of other learning differences, such as ADHD and dyslexia, but that there is "no awareness" of dyscalculia. Sylvia takes a broader view of this lack of awareness and understanding and believes this contributes to a lack of effective interventions for students. She recognized that while she was lucky to be diagnosed, her teachers were unable to help her learn math.

Research points to issues that contribute to a lack of awareness and understanding of dyscalculia. First, research in math-related learning differences is lagging behind that of other learning differences (Butterworth, 2019; Gersten et al., 2005). There is agreement among researchers that dyscalculia is a biological, brain-based learning difference (Butterworth, 2018; DeFina & Mosser, 2011; Knop & Chou, 2020; Szucs & Goswami, 2013). However, there is a lack of consensus on definitions, cognitive factors, and diagnostic criteria (Mazzocco & Myers, 2003; Szucs & Goswami, 2013). Even terminology is not agreed upon, with researchers using varied labels such as dyscalculia or developmental dyscalculia (Butterworth, 2019; Kosc, 1974), specific disorder of arithmetical skills (World Health Organization, 2009), specific learning disorder with impairment in mathematics (American Psychiatric Association, 2017), and mathematical learning disability or MD (Geary, 2004; Mazzocco & Myers, 2003). Importantly, without a thorough understanding of dyscalculia, practitioners find it difficult to identify effective teaching strategies (Butterworth et al., 2011). Additionally, there is little research on gifted students with dyscalculia (Knop & Chou, 2020), so the problems experienced by the participants in this study were largely unexamined.

Lesson 4: Strategies That Aid in Navigating Adult Challenges

The fourth theme that emerged from the findings was navigating challenges associated with dyscalculia as an adult. The participants demonstrated a range of experiences in this regard, from mild inconvenience to significant impact on their daily lives. The degree to which the participants have faced challenges in their adult lives seems related to the severity of their dyscalculia, as well as the level of independence they currently experience.

Most of James's memories of challenges with dyscalculia in school were related to calculation and recall of facts. He indicated that although he relies on computers to do math for him when needed, he feels he is able to understand any advanced concepts necessary for his work. Remembering meetings and balancing his checkbook were both identified as issues, but he has managed these problems by not worrying about missed meetings, and he avoids balancing his checkbook by always carrying a large balance. He believed that he has had "zero" problems in life related to math, though he acknowledged that he must use his fingers for even simple, single-digit calculations and that he still struggles with confidence related to math.

Amelia, in her late teens, and Louisa, in her mid-20s, are both living with parents and not yet fully responsible for themselves. They acknowledged they may feel differently once they are on their own, but for now their daily challenges as a result of dyscalculia have been minimal and mostly related to anxiety around performing math-related tasks, such as counting tips and change, telling time, and instances requiring calculation. Both individuals have relied on technology when math is needed: Amelia by using the cash register at work to calculate bills and change, and Louisa by using calculators, debit cards, and digital clocks. In spite of her discomfort, Louisa also learned that it's OK to ask for help and to accept that there are some things she cannot do.

Emma's and Sylvia's descriptions of their math understanding pointed to a more significant degree of challenge. Emma described being unable to subitize, struggling to calculate, difficulty gauging elapsed time and scheduling appointments, as well as not understanding measurement, distance, or directions. Sylvia described struggles with budgeting, elapsed time, scheduling, and measurement, and she shared that in eighth grade she was unable to show mastery of second-grade math content. She also described unexpected challenges, such as locating a departure gate at an airport and the impact of dyscalculia on her peer and family relationships and on her dating life.

Emma relied on some simple and commonplace strategies to navigate these challenges. For example, her husband took care of budgeting, and she relied on calculators and debit cards. Emma also worked hard to create strategies that allow her to be independent. She said she relies on a Time Timer, a common tool for time management in classrooms, to help her with following cooking times and taking care of various tasks. She learned to cook by sight and taste, without using measuring cups and spoons. Some of her strategies showed evidence of creative problem solving. She created playlists of different lengths to help her accomplish tasks in the appropriate length of time, and she added stickers to her speedometer to indicate position of the numbers in between those printed on the panel.

Sylvia's strategies for navigating challenges were largely based on getting help from others. For scheduling, she relied on following a routine and assistance from coworkers for double-checking her schedule. For financial matters, she depended on her mother for help. Like Louisa, Sylvia has learned to accept her limitations and become more comfortable with asking others for help.

As noted before, there are considerable gaps in the research on gifted individuals with dyscalculia (Knop & Chou, 2020). Studies on dyscalculia in adults are particularly difficult to find. A study by Vigna et al. (2022) provides evidence that difficulties in math do not resolve into adulthood among individuals with developmental dyscalculia (DD) and that their difficulties with math contribute to challenges with everyday tasks. The authors point to poor skills among adults with DD especially in the areas of time, measurement, and money. They also noted a negative impact on social and emotional well-being as early as primary school, with many of their participants reporting "tension, worry, frustration, anger, and psychosomatic symptoms . . . [and] feelings of frustration and guilt experienced when their difficulties during childhood were ascribed to lack of effort and motivation" (p. 8).

Revisiting the Research Questions

Coming back to the guiding research questions presented in Chapter 1, consider how your own thoughts, perspectives, and ideas connect to the findings shared in this chapter:

1. What are the academic, cognitive, social, emotional, and creative strengths of adults who have been identified as gifted and diagnosed with dyscalculia?
2. What academic, social, and extracurricular experiences of gifted adults with dyscalculia supported development of their strengths?
3. What academic, social, emotional, and extracurricular experiences of gifted adults with dyscalculia affected their ability to overcome academic, social, emotional, and cognitive challenges?
4. How do gifted adults with dyscalculia navigate math-related challenges in their personal and professional lives?

The lessons learned support conclusions that can be drawn in addressing these questions. In considering research question one, patterns of strengths were identified among the participants, namely in the areas of language arts, especially writing and communication; interpersonal skills; and creativity. All of the participants recognized these strengths in themselves in a variety of contexts, some from a very young age. For some of the participants, such as Sylvia and Louisa in writing and James for the creative thinking necessary for computer software design, these strengths were recognized before adulthood. For Emma and Amelia, their strengths were only identified at a later age through neuropsychological testing.

With regard to research question two, opportunities to develop strengths varied widely between participants and were in some ways related to whether or not strengths had been identified. James's recognition of his talent with computers in high school enabled him to be recruited for an internship that eventually became a job and jump-started his career in computer software design. Sylvia's middle school teacher provided an opportunity to develop her writing that became her first published book. Sylvia also participated in Odyssey of the Mind, which was her first opportunity to connect with like-minded peers as she developed her creative problem-solving skills. Sylvia, Louisa, Emma, and Amelia have all participated in performing arts in various ways, either by playing instruments (Emma and Amelia), singing (Amelia and Louisa), dancing (Amelia and Louisa), and participation in school theater and musical theater productions (Sylvia, Amelia, and Louisa). Additionally, Louisa had opportunities to take part in arts electives in high school in photography and graphic design, which set the stage for her now working to be a full-time artist.

Regarding research question three, while there was no obvious experience that enabled participants to overcome their challenges, they all demonstrated resilience, which helped them to cope with their struggles. In addition, they all had interesting insights about themselves and their perceptions, as well as a curiosity about their dual-gifted/learning difference nature, which has helped them to put their challenges into perspective.

Considering research question four, the participants demonstrated varying degrees of challenge in their personal and professional lives and developed a range of strategies to navigate those challenges. Some relied on simple strategies, such as using calculators, debit cards, digital clocks, and computers. Some relied on assistance from family and coworkers. Others have developed creative strategies to minimize the difficulties that dyscalculia presents, such as Emma's leveraging of her visual and auditory strengths in the ways that she relies on Time Timers and music playlists.

This chapter has highlighted the complex reality of being a gifted adult with dyscalculia—a reality characterized by a mix of notable strengths and significant challenges. Understanding twice-exceptionality requires more than recognizing difficulties; it calls for a holistic view that values the individual's unique talents alongside their learning differences, going beyond a deficit-only lens.

The findings emphasize the critical importance of early identification and a strength-based, talent-focused approach. Participants' experiences demonstrate how delayed or missed diagnoses and ineffective interventions contribute to frustration, anxiety, and difficulty in forming a positive self-concept. At the same time, recognition and development of strengths in areas such as language, creativity, and interpersonal skills promote motivation, resilience, and engagement.

In addition, the participants' adult lives demonstrate that dyscalculia's impact extends beyond the classroom, affecting daily functioning and requiring strategies to compensate. Their use of creative problem solving and reliance on support systems reflect the necessity of individualized approaches.

These insights point to an urgent need: moving from awareness to action. The lessons learned and shared here lay a foundation for the next chapter, which will focus on practical tips and strategies designed to empower gifted individuals with dyscalculia to navigate their challenges and thrive. Understanding the "why" is the first step—now it's time to explore the "how."

References

Al-Zoubi, S. M., & Al-Adawi, H. (2019). The effect of multiple intelligences strategies on academic achievement of students with mathematics learning disabilities. *Journal of Educational and Psychological Studies, 13*(1), 74–91. https://doi.org/10.24200/jeps.vol13iss1pp74-91

American Psychiatric Association. (2017). *Diagnostic and statistical manual of mental disorders* (5th ed., text rev.; DSM-5-TR). American Psychiatric Publishing.

Armstrong, T. (2010). *The power of neurodiversity: Unleashing the advantages of your differently wired brain.* Da Capo Lifelong Books.

Baum, S. M., Cooper, C. R., & Neu, T. W. (1997). Dual differentiation: An approach for meeting the curricular needs of gifted students with learning disabilities. *Psychology in the Schools, 34*(4), 305–317. https://doi.org/10.1002/(SICI)1520-6807(199710)34:4<305::AID-PITS6>3.0.CO;2-8

Baum, S. M., Renzulli, J. S., & Hébert, T. P. (1995). *The prism metaphor: A new paradigm for reversing underachievement*. Creative Learning Press.

Baum, S. M., Schader, R. M., & Hébert, T. P. (2014). Through a different lens: Reflecting on a strengths-based, talent-focused approach for twice-exceptional learners. *Gifted Child Quarterly, 58*(4), 311–327. https://doi.org/10.1177/0016986214547632

Baum, S. M., Schader, R. M., & Owen, S. V. (2017). *To be gifted and learning disabled: Strength-based strategies for helping twice-exceptional students with LD, ADHD, ASD, and more* (3rd ed.). Prufrock Press.

Butterworth, B. (2018). *Dyscalculia: From science to education*. Routledge. https://doi.org/10.4324/9781315115222

Butterworth, B. (2019). Dyscalculia: What's in a name? *ZDM—Mathematics Education, 51*, 965–971. https://doi.org/10.1007/s11858-019-01064-7

Butterworth, B., Varma, S., & Laurillard, D. (2011). Dyscalculia: From brain to education. *Science, 332*(6033), 1049–1053. https://doi.org/10.1126/science.1201536

Cain, W., O'Reilly, M., & Weir, K. (2019). Identification of twice-exceptional students: A qualitative study of school psychologists. *Contemporary School Psychology, 23*, 267–278. https://doi.org/10.1007/s40688-018-0186-3

Climie, E. A. (2015). Supporting children with attention-deficit/hyperactivity disorder with strengths-based approaches. *Canadian Psychology/Psychologie Canadienne, 56*(3), 258–265. https://doi.org/10.1037/cap0000030

DeFina, P. A., & Mosser, R. (2011). Mathematical learning disabilities and neuroscience: The need for clarity. *Applied Neuropsychology, 18*(2), 109–117. https://doi.org/10.1080/09084282.2011.595454

Eide, B. L., & Eide, F. F. (2012). *The dyslexic advantage: Unlocking the hidden potential of the dyslexic brain*. Plume.

Foley-Nicpon, M., Allmon, A., Sieck, B., & Stinson, R. D. (2013). Empirical investigation of twice-exceptionality: Where have we been and where are we going? *Gifted Child Quarterly, 57*(3), 169–180. https://doi.org/10.1177/0016986213490021

Geary, D. C. (2004). Mathematics and learning disabilities. *Journal of Learning Disabilities, 37*(1), 4–15. https://doi.org/10.1177/00222194040370010201

Gersten, R., Jordan, N. C., & Flojo, J. R. (2005). Early identification and interventions for students with mathematics difficulties. *Journal of Learning Disabilities, 38*(4), 293–304. https://doi.org/10.1177/00222194050380040301

Gilger, J. W., Pennington, B. F., & DeFries, J. C. (2008). A twin study of the etiology of comorbidity: Reading disability and attention-deficit/hyperactivity disorder. *Journal of Learning Disabilities*, 25(3), 231–240. https://doi.org/10.1177/002221949202500403

Karagiannakis, G., Baccaglini-Frank, A., & Papadatos, Y. (2014). Mathematical learning difficulties subtypes classification. *Frontiers in Human Neuroscience*, 8, Article 57. https://doi.org/10.3389/fnhum.2014.00057

Knop, B., & Chou, S. (2020). Twice-exceptional learners with dyscalculia: Identification, challenges, and strategies. *2e Newsletter*, 7(2), 8–15.

Kosc, L. (1974). Developmental dyscalculia. *Journal of Learning Disabilities*, 7(3), 164–177. https://doi.org/10.1177/002221947400700304

Lewis, K., & Lynn, M. (2018). Reframing dyscalculia: A positive approach to mathematical learning differences. *Mathematics Education Research Journal*, 30(2), 163–177. https://doi.org/10.1007/s13394-017-0220-7

Mazzocco, M. M. M., & Myers, G. F. (2003). Complexities in identifying and defining mathematics learning disability in the primary school-age years. *Annals of Dyslexia*, 53(1), 218–253. https://doi.org/10.1007/s11881-003-0011-7

Mundt, K. (2014). The need for professional development in identifying twice-exceptional learners. *Gifted Child Today*, 37(4), 219–225. https://doi.org/10.1177/1076217514544024

Olenchak, F. R. (1995). Effects of talent search programming on the social self-concept of gifted learning-disabled students. *Roeper Review*, 17(3), 173–176. https://doi.org/10.1080/02783199509553657

Olenchak, F. R. (2009). Students with disabilities and giftedness: A promising interface. In L. V. Shavinina (Ed.), *International handbook on giftedness* (pp. 161–173). Springer. https://doi.org/10.1007/978-1-4020-6162-2_11

Ottone-Cross, K., Boazman, J., & Owens, D. (2016). The twice-exceptional paradox: A qualitative study of the experiences of gifted students with ADHD. *Gifted Child Today*, 39(4), 207–214. https://doi.org/10.1177/1076217516654086

Peterson, C. (2009). *Pursuing the good life: 100 reflections on positive psychology*. Oxford University Press.

Rappolt-Schlichtmann, G., Boucher, A. R., & Evans, M. (2018). From deficit remediation to capacity building: Learning to enable rather than disable students with dyslexia. *Language, Speech & Hearing Services in Schools (Online)*, 49(4), 864–874. https://doi.org/10.1044/2018_LSHSS-DYSLC-18-0031

Reis, S. M., Baum, S. M., & Burke, E. (2014). An operational definition of twice-exceptional learners: Implications and applications. *Gifted Child Quarterly, 58*(3), 217–230. https://doi.org/10.1177/0016986214534976

Schneps, M. (2014). The advantages of dyslexia. *Scientific American Mind, 26*(1), 24-25. https://www.scientificamerican.com/article/the-advantages-of-dyslexia/

Seligman, M. E. P., & Csikszentmihalyi, M. (2000). Positive psychology: An introduction. *American Psychologist, 55*(1), 5–14. https://doi.org/10.1037/0003-066X.55.1.5

Szucs, D., & Goswami, U. (2013). Developmental dyscalculia: Fresh perspectives. *Trends in Neuroscience and Education, 2*(2), 33–37. https://doi.org/10.1016/j.tine.2013.06.004

Vigna, D., Valenti, M., & Pievani, T. (2022). Developmental dyscalculia in adults: An exploratory study on everyday impact. *Annals of Dyslexia, 72*, 1–17. https://doi.org/10.1007/s11881-021-00236-2

World Health Organization. (2009). *International statistical classification of diseases and related health problems* (10th rev.) (ICD-10). WHO Press.

Wright, B. (2013). *Autism and creativity: Is there a link between autism in the family and creativity?* Psychology Press.

6
Tips, Strategies, and Suggestions

Hopefully, the stories and information shared up to this point have been illuminating; however, if you're a parent or a teacher of a dyscalculic person, or if you are struggling with dyscalculia yourself, you may be asking, OK, now what? What can we do? This chapter presents practical suggestions for a variety of contexts, pulled from personal experience with dyscalculic students, the experiences of others who have found success working with individuals with dyscalculia, and the study participants themselves.

What NOT to Do

Before getting started with what does work, it is important to consider what does *not* work.

"Just Try Harder"

Louisa often spoke about her frustration with being made to feel that she was just lazy and that putting more effort into her math work would solve the problem. When she transferred to her boarding school, she said the reaction to her math struggles was along the lines of "This is a smart kid and she's not trying hard enough. She's lazy." She had a similar experience when she attempted math courses at a community college. She told those professors, "I truly don't understand that," and their response was "Try harder."

Louisa recognized at a fairly young age that she needed to be taught math in a different way, but lack of understanding about dyscalculia and lack of a formal diagnosis prevented her from getting what she needed. She felt immense relief once she was finally diagnosed, sharing, "[They] gave it a name, and [then] nobody [was] looking at me like I'm lazy for not trying hard enough."

Sylvia also recounted how trying harder was a fruitless endeavor for her. She shared stories of her mother's tireless efforts to help her learn math facts with no results. She was lucky to have a math teacher in middle school who recognized that for her, effort did not equal outcome. To revisit a quote shared earlier, he said he'd "never seen anyone work so hard and fail so much."

A colorblind analogy has helped some students, parents, and teachers understand the difficulties of learning math with dyscalculia (Butterworth, 2005). A totally colorblind person can learn strategies to navigate situations where being able to see colors is important—traffic lights, for example. However, no amount of effort is going to make that colorblind person see the red, yellow, and green of the traffic light in the way that someone with typical color vision will see, and suggesting they just try harder to see those colors is frustrating and absurd.

Dyscalculia is a cognitive difference. Mathematical skills and concepts will be processed in ways that are different from a neurotypical person. Being told to just try harder, for most individuals, will be largely ineffective and can have negative emotional, social, and academic consequences, as happened with many of the study participants.

"You Just Need More Practice"

Similar to trying harder, giving more practice without the necessary support can be frustrating and demoralizing. Emma shared stories about being given extra work to do. When asked what teachers did to help her, she said, "mostly, it was like more math was assigned to me. I [would] get more worksheets and more math like, 'Oh, you're bad at this so here, do more of it. Have more of it to do at home and that'll help you.'" Emma was perplexed by this approach and didn't understand how anyone thought that extra worksheets would improve her understanding.

Emma and Louisa both compared math to learning a foreign language, and this analogy works here. Practice is essential to mastering a foreign language; however, with no understanding of the foundations of a language, extra verb conjugation worksheets are unlikely to increase your fluency and may just sour your attitude about learning the language. Extra practice can be helpful to address challenges of dyscalculia, but only when used in a productive way, which will be addressed later in this chapter.

"You Can Do It, It's Easy"

Well-meaning teachers and parents use this line with the best of intentions—to provide encouragement and be a cheerleader for a struggling student. Everyone benefits from encouragement, but when a student is already struggling with self-efficacy, being told that something that is very hard for them is "easy" only adds to confusion and feelings of incompetence.

James and Louisa both spoke passionately about often feeling stupid and being confused as to why something that others seemed able to do without a problem was so frustratingly hard for them. The word stupid came up numerous times in both of their interviews.

James: "I really struggled with the idea that I wasn't stupid."

"I thought . . . there's a level of stupid that I must be. And it just shocked me that I could not learn it."

Louisa: "Why do I feel smart and stupid at the same time? . . . It was just really frustrating."

"I would feel this sort of impostor syndrome . . . this person thinks I'm smart, but after they're going to know that I'm not . . . so it's this anxiety about feeling like people are going to think I'm stupid."

"I was crying to [my therapist], saying, sometimes I feel so stupid. Am I stupid?"

"Sometimes on a bad day, I'm thinking, I'm stupid. I think I'm like a literal idiot or something."

"When I'm met with my weaknesses, [I feel like] I'm so stupid and [if] I'm so smart, why can't I do that?"

Understanding Your Brain

Direct, honest conversation about everyone's brains being different and processing things in different ways is essential. Due to a concern about labels and the stigma often associated with disabilities of all kinds, many parents are understandably hesitant about seeking a formal diagnosis or disclosing a diagnosed learning disability to their child or their child's teachers. However, awareness and understanding of how your brain works support self-awareness and a positive self-concept, which can lead to the development of self-advocacy skills and improve the chances of finding effective learning strategies. For teachers of children who struggle, knowing about a diagnosis gives them better tools and understanding and gives teachers a better chance of finding the most effective ways to teach. And for the students themselves, most children are keenly aware about differences in the classroom, so in the absence of that crucial information, many just assume they are stupid.

Individuals with dyscalculia need to understand that their brains process numbers and math differently, and they need to know what their strengths are. In their interviews, the depth of the shame and confusion that the participants felt was palpable. If someone had explained to them how their brains are different and helped them to see their strengths, that would have gone a long way to helping them develop a more positive sense of self and to understand that they are not stupid or broken but just different.

One of the students referenced in the introduction to this book was Eloise, a brilliant fourth-grade student who was diagnosed with dyscalculia. Her parents were worried about the negative impact of a label and requested that teachers not share with her that she had a learning difference. She was smart enough to know that something that was easy for her classmates was very hard for her. Her parents were well meaning and just wanted what was best for her, but without information that would explain her struggles, Eloise's conclusion was that she was just stupid.

Starting With Strengths

Connect to strengths and interests as much as possible! For another student, Andrew, referenced in the introduction, his dyscalculia was severe. He was working many years below grade level in math and struggling with essential foundational skills and concepts, like accurate counting of objects in the single digits and place value of even three- and four-digit numbers. This student really struggled to manage his emotions when introduced to new concepts and skills. He was talented and highly interested in music, so when he was introduced to fractions concepts in the context of rhythmic notation in music (whole notes, half notes, quarter notes, etc.), he showed a better understanding of new material than he usually did. By connecting something unfamiliar and hard with something familiar and easy, he was able to make sense of the new material. In addition, there was none of the frustration he typically demonstrated with new content, and he actually enjoyed it.

Research supports a strength-based, talent-focused approach as the most effective teaching practice for twice-exceptional students (Baum et al., 2017). Numerous benefits have been identified not only for 2e students but for all students, including stronger social relationships, development of expertise in talent areas, improved academic achievement, development of a positive self-concept, and an increase in the ability to navigate social, emotional, and cognitive challenges (Baum et al., 1995, 2014, 2017; Olenchak, 2009; Reis et al., 2014). Studies on twice-exceptional students show that an emphasis on strengths, paired with a de-emphasis on deficits, results in engaged and successful students who have more conspicuous gifted characteristics (Reis et al., 2014).

James, Sylvia, and Louisa, who were recognized for their strengths from a younger age, were better able to see themselves as intelligent and capable in spite of their challenges. Emma and Amelia, however, struggled to see themselves as gifted, even in their strength areas, in spite of formal identification and clear evidence.

Strengths and interests can be leveraged to tackle challenges; however, strengths and interests should also be nurtured, encouraged, and celebrated for their own sake and not just as tools to do the hard things. A strong word of caution here: leveraging a strength or interest area in every situation where a student struggles can be tempting; however, there is a very real risk of the student feeling a loss of ownership over skills, topics, and activities that may have felt like their only safe space.

Research shows that it is essential to view strengths and interests as two sides of the same coin: they can be highly effective as a support for challenges AND they should be nurtured and valued in their own right. Additionally, overuse of a student's strength areas as remediation has the potential for diminishing intrinsic motivation and personal fulfillment from participating in those activities or topics. It can feel like a co-opting of an individual's comfort zone, which negatively affects joy, self-expression, sense of identity, and emotional safety (Baum et al., 2015)

Compensatory Strategies for Teaching, Learning, and Living

Oftentimes, a neurotypical parent or teacher will, with the best of intentions, try to impose a strategy that makes perfect sense for a neurotypical brain, but neurotypical thinking doesn't always make sense for a neurodivergent brain. On the flip side of that, compensatory strategies that someone with dyscalculia comes up with may be discouraged because they seem inefficient or even nonsensical to a neurotypical person. For example, a 50-year old dyscalculic woman, who was not part of the study, struggles with budgeting. To keep track of her spending, she's devised a system that involves two checking accounts and shuffling money back and forth between the two to pay her bills and minimize the chances of overdrawing on her account. Her father, a retired accountant, has tried to get her to use a more efficient system, but she's not able to manage her money independently with his system. Hers is a cumbersome approach, and it's not perfect, but it works well for her, because it makes sense to her.

Everyone is unique, and what works wonders for someone may not be effective for others. Experiment! Try different strategies. Find something that works for *that* unique brain. And remember that ownership of strategies is important. The individual who needs support should always be involved in discussions about strategies and/or classroom accommodations. That being said, following are some strategies applicable to a variety of contexts that some may find beneficial. These suggestions come from the author's own teaching experience and informal experimentation; however, many are closely aligned with suggestions found in the work of respected dyscalculia researchers and authors, such as Brian Butterworth, Steve Chinn, and Paul Moorcraft. See Table 6.1 later in the chapter for suggested resources that include their work.

For Math Teachers (or Math-Adjacent Subjects, Like Chemistry, for Example)

Dyscalculic students often struggle to learn math in the traditional ways, so priorities in teaching may need to be adjusted for these students, and progress will look different. Keep these three ideas in mind: minimize anxiety as much as possible; allow students to move at their own pace of readiness; and situate math learning in concrete, relevant, and real-world contexts. An anxious brain cannot take in and retain new information, so anxiety creates a slippery slope, where the student doesn't understand, becomes stressed about not understanding, is unable to learn because stress is affecting their ability to learn, and then anxiety increases, and the spiral continues as the student falls further behind. Attention to readiness and real-world contexts can also serve to alleviate stress. Math is often cumulative in

TABLE 6.1 Recommended resources for more information

Multisensory math

Zoid and Company https://zoidandcompany.com/	Website of Dr. Rachel McAnallen, which includes a list of her available workshops (some including links to scripted lessons) and a wide variety of manipulatives.
Multisensory Math https://www.multisensorymath.com/	Website with information about Marilyn Zecher, multisensory math, workshop information, and other information.
Made for Math https://madeformath.com/	An online tutoring service, based on the work of Marilyn Zecher, specializing in multisensory math approaches for students with learning differences that affect math.

Researchers and websites with a specific focus on dyscalculia

Brian Butterworth https://brian-butterworth.com/	Website of a neuroscientist who is a leading researcher in dyscalculia. Includes valuable information about dyscalculia, his research, and many resources. Brian Butterworth also has many engaging presentations that are accessible for a wide audience posted on YouTube.
The Dyscalculia Association http://www.dyscalculiaassociation.uk/	A UK-based website created by Steve Chinn and Judy Hornigold that contains a wealth of valuable information about dyscalculia, training courses for teachers, and links to plenty of resources, including websites, videos, articles, books, and more.
Steve Chinn https://www.stevechinn.co.uk/	Considerable background information about dyscalculia, including a breakdown of the research on dyscalculia at different grade levels, diagnostic information, checklists of characteristics, links to his books and articles, and a lengthy section on math anxiety.

Websites with a specific focus on twice-exceptionality

The 2e Center for Research and Professional Development www.2ecenter.org	Offers a variety of articles and other resources and is accessible for parents and nonspecialists, as well as gifted and 2e educators and researchers.

The Strength-Based Assessment Lab at Bridges Graduate School of Cognitive Diversity in Education https://strength-based-assessment-lab.my.canva.site/	Led by Dr. Jade Rivera, the Lab focuses on empowering students, families, and educators by identifying and nurturing neurodivergent children's strengths and interests. Through collaborative assessments, the Lab helps create personalized learning environments and strength-based individualized education program (IEP) goals—shifting the focus from deficits to assets and providing practical strategies for caregivers and educators to support twice-exceptional learners.

Books

Baum, S. M., Schader, R., & Owen, S. (2017). *To be gifted and learning disabled: Strength-based strategies for helping twice-exceptional students with LD, ADHD, and more*. Prufrock Press.

Butterworth, B. (2019). *Dyscalculia: From science to education*. Routledge.

Chinn, S., & Ashcroft, R. (2017). *Mathematics for dyslexics and dyscalculics: A teaching handbook*. Wiley Blackwell.

Moorcraft, P. (2014). *It just doesn't add up: Explaining dyscalculia and overcoming number problems for children and adults*. Tarquin.

nature, so moving ahead before a student is confident in the skills and concepts needed for the next level sets that student up for failure and more anxiety. As for concrete, relevant, and real-world contexts, there is plenty of research to support this approach.

With this guiding framework in mind, following is an exploration of a variety of strategies and instructional approaches that have demonstrated potential for success with dyscalculic students.

Many experts have published and shared their own strategies, some of whom will be referenced later in this chapter. The tips, strategies, and suggestions you find here—though there will be overlap with best practices supported by other researchers—stem from conclusions drawn from my own experiences teaching students with dyscalculia, with connections drawn to the stories of the study participants when warranted.

Alleviating Math Anxiety

As noted earlier, anxiety is a significant roadblock to learning. When a student feels threatened, unsafe, misunderstood, or worried, the effect is that the "stress and anxiety short circuit neural pathways . . . [and] halt the processes of reasoning, memory, self- and impulse-control—the very skills that are essential to successful learning" (Baum et al., 2017). So how does a teacher create a psychologically safe learning environment, where students who tend to feel anxious don't need to go into survival mode to get through a math class?

Play can be a great way to approach learning, and many students have found success through math games; however, if other needs aren't being met, sometimes a math game can heighten anxiety and cause a struggling student to feel exposed. While the following strategies, approaches, and suggestions may not explicitly address anxiety, many of them have the benefit of alleviating anxiety by addressing underlying challenges.

An Emphasis on Conceptual Understanding Over Memorizing Algorithms

Many dyscalculic students struggle with remembering math facts and procedures. If a student understands WHY something works the way it does, then they can use logical reasoning and problem solving to figure it out (or figure out a reasonable solution) if they can't remember the facts or the steps. Related to that, it's helpful to focus on process and understanding over finding the correct solution. Dr. Rachel McAnallen, known as Ms. Math, has been an influential model for many math teachers due to her expertise in math anxiety and her emphasis on prioritizing conceptual understanding. A fun, low-stakes, and effective strategy she encourages is to give a math problem, then give the answer before students work the problem. Tell the students that the right answer isn't important; instead, they should prove that the given answer is correct. This strategy takes the pressure off of finding the answer and helps students really think through what is happening and why.

Error analysis is also a great tool for developing conceptual understanding. If a student is able to find out *why* their work is wrong, that shows deeper understanding than getting the answer right the first time. If the answer was correct, maybe they understand the problem, or maybe they're just good at following the algorithm but don't know what's happening. If a student can do error analysis, they understand what's going on. Error analysis is a fantastic tool, because it encourages deep thinking and conceptual understanding, and because it also normalizes mistakes and makes them a critical part of learning. Depending on the severity of an individual's dyscalculia, however, that does have the potential to be frustrating, so proceed with caution and be prepared to provide necessary scaffolding. In general, however, normalizing mistakes and modeling productive failure support a classroom environment where all students feel free to make mistakes without stress or worry.

"Little and Often"
Targeted, guided repetition on concepts and skills, what the Dyscalculia Association calls the "little and often" approach, is essential. This is not to be confused with extra practice time, or more work, or more problems to solve. As Emma shared from her experiences, extra practice without understanding or appropriate support is just frustrating and ineffective.

What this might look like is mini-lessons at the beginning of each session that serve as quick reviews and/or reteaching of previously taught material. The goal is for students to not just learn the material but to be continually exposed to it over time. Research shows that spaced repetition, or distributed practice, greatly improves retention of information and skills (Rohrer & Taylor, 2006). Andrew, the student with severe dyscalculia, required frequent repetition to come anywhere near showing mastery of concepts and skills. And then, once he could show independence with that concept or skill, he would lose what progress he had made if he was not given near-daily opportunities to review and relearn. Over time, Andrew made great progress with this approach, progressing from standardized math scores in single-digit percentiles to around the 50th percentile one year later.

A little and often approach requires a great deal of patience, an ability to gauge a student's readiness to move forward, and a willingness to move at the pace of the student. In a typical classroom, this strategy would be extremely difficult—this is more suited to one-on-one or small-group instruction, as would be found in tutoring or small-group pull-out programs, such as Andrew's.

Number Flexibility: An Emphasis on Place Value Concepts and Number Sense

Another beneficial strategy for dyscalculic students is beginning each math class with a number flexibility warm-up. This activity involves decomposing and partitioning a given number, which are similar tasks that involve breaking up a number into parts. The parts can be partitioned by breaking up a number by digit and place value, for example, $253 = 200 + 50 + 3$. Or a number can be decomposed into other parts, for example, $10 = 5 + 5$ or $10 = 12 - 2$.

In this whole-group warm-up activity, another activity from Rachel McAnallen, students are given a number, and they offer as many ways as possible to represent that number. For example, given 25, students could offer $20 + 5$, or $10 + 10 + 5$, or $28 - 3$, or 5×5, or $50 \div 2$, or many other ways. There are a few reasons why this is a positive and productive activity: it builds number sense in a playful way; it helps to develop place value concepts; it allows students to work at their own level (struggling students tend to give a lot of addition, but advanced students can think about fractions, or longer number sentences with multiple operations, which then has the added bonus of providing a relevant way to teach order of operations with mixed operation number sentences); and it provides an opportunity to identify patterns that connect to multiplication or division ($5 + 5 + 5 + 5 + 5$ is the same as 5×5) or other interesting patterns that reveal something about how numbers work (like $25 + 0$, $24 + 1$, $23 + 2$, $22 + 3$, etc.). Students tend to really enjoy this warm-up, because they can make it as easy or hard for themselves as they want to, and even the ones who are trying to make it easy still have to think it through to figure out what easy is, which helps them all with understanding numbers a little better.

A heavy focus on place value, number sense, and conceptual understanding is highly beneficial for struggling math students, and once students are comfortable with number flexibility activities, they can then use that skill to support work with addition, subtraction, multiplication, and division. This strategy is once again a nod to Rachel McAnallen work. Her methods for teaching the four basic operations allow the student some choice in how they set up a problem, because they can decide how to decompose or partition a number, and they can choose a number that's easier for them to work with. For example, if it's difficult and stressful for a student to add 7, then they can choose to use $5 + 2$ instead, because 5 and 2 are much more "friendly." These are not efficient methods for doing multidigit operations, but students will build understanding of place value and improve their number sense. In fact, all students, dyscalculic or not, can benefit from learning these methods before moving on to standard algorithms, because they will really understand what is happening in a problem.

Multisensory Teaching Strategies

A multisensory approach to math is a research-supported approach that has been shown to be highly effective for many struggling students. Research demonstrates that tapping into multiple senses creates more and stronger connections in the brain to support learning and memory (Taneja & Sankhian, 2019). Many teachers and specialists support the use of multisensory math, which has developed over the years thanks to the work of Marilyn Zecher and is based on Orton-Gillingham teaching methods. Some of the foundations of a multisensory approach are the use of manipulatives and an emphasis on conceptual understanding. Resources for more information on multisensory math are included in Table 6.1.

A note about counting on fingers: manipulatives have become an increasingly common tool in math classrooms because teachers understand their value. What about fingers as manipulatives? Many dedicated and well-intentioned teachers discourage counting on fingers, but fingers, for many, are an intuitive tool for counting. Telling students who have difficulty learning math facts not to count on their fingers does not support automaticity of math facts. Often, the student just hides their hands under the desk, which can lead to feelings of shame and embarrassment. Normalizing and modeling counting with fingers can minimize anxiety and create a psychologically safe environment for students, even as they continue to work toward fluency in math facts.

Classroom Accommodations

Accommodations are very important, and in my experience, a lot of great teachers tend to push back against students being allowed to use calculators or multiplication facts charts. It's a reasonable concern—they know that math facts automaticity frees up mental energy to do the "real" work of math. However, for students who struggle to memorize math facts, as many with dyscalculia do (as well as those with dyslexia, attention deficit hyperactivity disorder [ADHD], and working memory deficits), not allowing a calculator puts up an unnecessary barrier. They need the calculator to be able to access the higher-level material.

Appropriate accommodations can vary greatly from student to student, depending on the needs of the individual. Examples of some common accommodations include:

- Use of a calculator, especially when calculating is not what's being assessed
- Use of number lines and/or facts sheets

- Use of checklists to aid memory (e.g., steps for an algorithm or list of formulas)
- Additional time for assignments and tests
- A separate, quiet space with minimal distractions for testing
- Frequent checks for understanding
- Use of graph paper to aid in place value alignment for vertical calculations
- Adjusted test formatting (fewer problems per page, more open space)

It's worth repeating that what works for one person doesn't always work for another and also that each person's experience with and impact from dyscalculia will be different. Therefore, it's important to work closely with teachers, psychologists, and the student to identify what accommodations are most appropriate for the individual. Even when used with fidelity, accommodations aren't intended to make the work easy, but they should minimize or eliminate barriers to success.

Suggested Resources

Strategies for teaching and learning is a big topic—much larger than can be comfortably addressed in a single chapter. For a deeper dive, consider the resources found in Table 6.1.

Navigating Adulthood

Dyscalculic children will grow up into dyscalculic adults. Those with little understanding of dyscalculia may say, "No problem! You don't have to worry about math classes anymore!" However, the impact of dyscalculia goes beyond the math classroom. While it may seem obvious that a dyscalculic person would have difficulty with money (including shopping and money management), dyscalculic individuals also commonly struggle with time, measurement, scheduling, driving, following directions, cooking, pursuing careers, interpersonal relationships, mental health, and more. In addition, dyscalculia can have significant negative impacts on lifetime earnings potential and can create roadblocks for educational advancement (Butterworth, 2019).

So in the face of these challenges, how can a dyscalculic adult achieve a fulfilling, independent life? As emphasized earlier in this chapter, everyone is unique, and no strategy will be equally effective for everyone. Just as with teaching and learning strategies, ways of navigating the challenges of adult life will require experimentation to find what works for the individual. Following is a summary of suggested strategies and tools, including some that the study participants found to be effective.

Money
Adult responsibilities dealing with money are probably the most obvious area where support would be needed; challenges can involve a wide range of money-related situations, such as negotiating a salary and benefits, savings and investment, balancing a checkbook, budgeting, calculating tips, making purchases, and more. Some suggestions for managing money-related situations include:

- Use credit cards and debit cards instead of cash *(Amelia, Louisa)*.
- Take advantage of technology, like smart phones and computers, to do calculations for you *(James, Amelia)*.
- Recruit partners, siblings, or parents to provide support with managing finances *(Emma, Sylvia)*.
- If your finances allow, carry a large checking account balance to avoid overdrawing *(James)*.
- Hire a trustworthy financial advisor for long-term planning and investment advice.
- Explore apps for a variety of money-related tasks: tips, budgets, etc.

Schedules, Routines, and Keeping Track of Time
Calendars and schedules can be a challenge, and the most effective strategies will likely depend on your learning preferences and organizational style.

- At work, have a trusted colleague double-check your schedule for errors *(Sylvia)*.

- Use visual timers to gauge the passage of time or to complete routine tasks (*Emma*).
- Create playlists of different lengths of time to help with time management (*Emma*).
- Create familiar routines (*Sylvia*).
- Use physical calendars or digital calendar apps for scheduling.

In the Kitchen

Shopping for and preparing food involve a lot of math, including the need to understand quantities, volume, fractions, oven temperatures, and cooking times.

- Use visual timers (*Emma*) or digital timers.
- Consider an oven with a digital temperature display.
- Experiment and build confidence cooking by sight and taste, rather than by using specific measurements (*Emma*).
- Use a meal planning app that generates a grocery list for you.
- Look for measuring cup and spoon sets with more pieces to allow matching the measurement in the recipe to the measurement printed on the cup or spoon and eliminate the need to figure out how many of one fraction is needed to make another.

Driving and Directions

For dyscalculics who struggle with understanding speed limits and with directions, including reading maps and distinguishing left from right, driving can be daunting.

- Customize your speedometer with stickers to indicate numbers not printed (*Emma*).
- Follow the flow of traffic to gauge your speed (*Emma*).
- Use landmarks instead of directional words for navigating (*Emma*).
- Use voice-guided global positioning system (GPS) apps.
- For navigating public transportation, use apps designed for that purpose, which can provide detailed information about stops and transfers.

Mental Health
Sylvia emphasized the importance of being mindful of stress levels and finding time for self-care and shared that dyscalculia-related challenges were harder to manage when anxiety increases. Make time to do things that keep you healthy and bring you joy and calm, such as:

- Get adequate sleep.
- Find time for exercise that works for you and makes you feel good.
- Make time for rest and relaxation.
- Pursue hobbies and interests.
- Try meditation.
- Get out in nature.
- Connect with friends and family.
- Develop a support system of people you can rely on when you are struggling.

Asking for Help
Sylvia and Louisa both noted a growing awareness into adulthood of the acceptability of just asking someone for help, with Sylvia expressing that she would have been mortified to ask for help when she was younger but feels more comfortable doing so now.

Niche Construction

Thomas Armstrong (2012, 2021) adapted earlier theories of biological evolution through an educational and psychological lens. In these contexts, niche construction applies to the idea of creating environments that are more aligned with an individual's strengths, interests, and neurological profile, which fits very well with a strength-based approach. Rather than trying to fix what's wrong to better fit in, the goal is to craft environments where the individual can thrive. In a neurotypical world, this can feel like a difficult task; however, creating an ideal environment can be as simple as asking these questions: *What are your passions? What sparks your curiosity? Under what circumstances do you feel you are your best self? When have you felt confident and capable? What strengths do you have, including nonacademic strengths?*

When niche construction is applied, individuals find more opportunities to be more engaged and motivated and to develop a stronger and more positive sense of self. An added benefit is that niche construction doesn't apply only to educational contexts but can also help shape career paths that are more likely to be fulfilling. However, there is an important caveat—niche construction should not be interpreted to mean that a 2e dyscalculic person is limited only to those fields that avoid math and play to their strengths. Do what makes you happy and fulfilled. A fascinating example of this at play is found in an article cowritten by a statistics major with dyscalculia (Lewis & Lynn, 2018). If statistics is your passion and you are motivated to succeed, then pursue it!

Conclusion

While dyscalculia can pose significant challenges across a variety of contexts—school, home, the workplace, relationships, and more—this chapter illustrates that a strength-based approach, coupled with effective strategies, can support students in developing confidence and creating a place for themselves where they are more likely to thrive. Beyond an educational context, understanding the broad impact of dyscalculia on adult life highlights the importance of appropriate support, problem solving, self-advocacy, and full recognition of strengths and talents. With patience, creativity, respectful understanding, and a focus on what they do best, individuals with dyscalculia can thrive in their learning and in their lives.

References

The 2e Center for Research and Professional Development. (n.d.). *The 2e Center*. https://www.2ecenter.org/

Armstrong, T. (2012). *Neurodiversity in the classroom: Strength-based strategies to help students with special needs succeed in school and life*. ASCD.

Armstrong, T. (2021). *The power of neurodiversity: Unleashing the advantages of your differently wired brain* (Updated ed.). Da Capo Lifelong Books.

Baum, S. M., Owen, S. V., & Dixon, J. (1995). *To be gifted and learning disabled: From identification to practical intervention strategies.* Creative Learning Press.

Baum, S. M., Schader, R. M., & Hébert, T. P. (2014). Through a different lens: Reflecting on a strengths-based, talent-focused approach for twice-exceptional learners. *Gifted Child Quarterly, 58*(4), 311–327. https://doi.org/10.1177/0016986214547632

Baum, S. M., Schader, R. M., & Hébert, T. P. (2017). The prism model: A new paradigm for identifying and nurturing talent in students with special needs. *Roeper Review, 39*(3), 124–138. https://doi.org/10.1080/02783193.2017.1318028

Baum, S. M., Schader, R. M., Hébert, T. P., & Owen, S. V. (2015). A strength-based approach for 2e students: Enhancing potential and possibilities. *Gifted Child Today, 38*(4), 192–201. https://doi.org/10.1177/1076217515597275

Butterworth, B. (2005). The development of arithmetical abilities. *Journal of Child Psychology and Psychiatry, 46*(1), 3–18. https://doi.org/10.1111/j.1469-7610.2004.00374.x

Butterworth, B. (2019). *Dyscalculia: From science to education.* Routledge.

Butterworth, B. (n.d.). *Brian Butterworth.* https://brian-butterworth.com/

Chinn, S. (n.d.). *Steve Chinn.* https://www.stevechinn.co.uk/

Chinn, S., & Ashcroft, R. (2017). *Mathematics for dyslexics and dyscalculics: A teaching handbook.* Wiley Blackwell.

The Dyscalculia Association. (n.d.). *The Dyscalculia Association.* http://www.dyscalculiaassociation.uk/

Lewis, K. E., & Lynn, D. M. (2018). Against the odds: Insights from a statistician with dyscalculia. *Education Sciences, 8*(63), 1–10. https://doi.org/10.3390/educsci8020063

Made for Math. (n.d.). *Made for Math.* https://madeformath.com/

Moorcraft, P. (2014). *It just doesn't add up: Explaining dyscalculia and overcoming number problems for children and adults.* Tarquin.

Multisensory Math. (n.d.). *Multisensory Math.* https://www.multisensorymath.com/

Olenchak, F. R. (2009). Effects of talent-focused education on the social self-concept of students with academic learning disabilities. *Gifted Child Quarterly, 53*(4), 280–288. https://doi.org/10.1177/0016986209346942

Reis, S. M., Baum, S. M., & Burke, E. (2014). An operational definition of twice-exceptional learners: Implications and applications. *Gifted Child Quarterly*, *58*(3), 217–230. https://doi.org/10.1177/0016986214534976

Rohrer, D., & Taylor, K. (2006). The effects of overlearning and distributed practice on the retention of mathematics knowledge. *Applied Cognitive Psychology*, *20*(9), 1209–1224. https://doi.org/10.1002/acp.1266

Strength-Based Assessment Lab. (n.d.). *Strength-Based Assessment Lab at Bridges Graduate School of Cognitive Diversity in Education*. https://strength-based-assessment-lab.my.canva.site/

Taneja, K. K., & Sankhian, A. (2019). Effect of multi-sensory approach on performance in mathematics at primary level. *The Educational Beacon*, *8*, 93–101.

Zoid and Company. (n.d.). *Zoid and Company*. https://zoidandcompany.com/

7

Conclusion

As this book draws to a close, it is important to reflect not only on what was discovered but also on what remains to be done. While the rich personal stories of the participants shine a spotlight on significant patterns and insights, the research process itself comes with limitations. This chapter begins by acknowledging those limitations and then shifts toward practical recommendations for educators, researchers, and advocates. Rooted in both participant voices and a strength-based perspective, these recommendations serve to inform, inspire, and empower. The chapter includes a call to action, encouraging readers to take meaningful steps toward greater awareness, empathy, and equity for gifted individuals with dyscalculia. Finally, the chapter, and the book, closes with an expression of gratitude for the contributions of the study participants and hopes for positive change to come.

Limitations

As with much research, there were a few limitations that may have affected this study and its conclusions, the first of which is researcher bias. Researcher bias risks "allowing one's personal views and perspectives to affect how data are interpreted" (Johnson, 2008, p. 284). This was addressed in a straightforward manner by simply being aware of biases and engaging in intentional self-reflection throughout the process, what in

DOI: 10.4324/9781003527800-7

research terms would be called reflexivity. Another strategy to address potential bias was addressed by using low-inference descriptors—direct quotes and language that are close to the participants' language—so there is less chance of misinterpreting the participants' experiences and viewpoints.

Interpretive validity deals with "the degree to which the research participants' viewpoints, thoughts, feelings, intentions, and experiences are accurately understood by the qualitative researcher and portrayed in the research report" (Johnson, 2008, p. 285). This was addressed through the use of low-inference descriptors (noted earlier), as well as member checking. Having participants verify their language and thoughts ensured an accurate portrayal of their experiences and feelings.

Recruitment for the study was a challenge, resulting in a small sample size, although data saturation was achieved with the participants involved in the study. Self-selection bias may affect the validity of this study because the experiences of those who choose to participate may not be representative of the general population of gifted adults with dyscalculia. Awareness of this issue could serve to bring in more participants for future studies.

Recommendations for Educators and Higher Education

This study offers a number of recommendations for educators and higher education programs that would serve to benefit twice-exceptional students with dyscalculia. First, teacher training programs in higher education must commit to improving awareness of and strategies for working with twice-exceptional students and students with dyscalculia. An understanding and awareness of this learning difference will enable teachers to recognize signs of dyscalculia and recommend evaluation to support earlier diagnosis and intervention. Teachers must also be trained to be aware of and recognize co-occurring conditions along with the additional complexities that a student with multiple learning differences presents. Additionally, improved understanding of the needs of twice-exceptional students, especially from a strength-based, talent-focused perspective, would allow educators to better meet those needs and to cultivate a student's strengths while supporting deficits.

In addition to increasing their awareness and understanding of dyscalculia and twice-exceptional learners, teachers must commit to finding new tools for teaching struggling math students that follow research-based best practices and serve to support math learning for these students. Gifted students with dyscalculia need alternative strategies for math learning, while also receiving appropriate levels of challenge that match their intellectual potential. Teachers must also develop an understanding of the impact of stress on learning and should work to minimize stress as much as possible in the math classroom.

Recommendations for Further Research

Looking back to the existing research, there are multiple areas with gaps. First, more research is needed toward developing a consensus of definitions and diagnostic criteria for dyscalculia. This will ensure that future research is focused on dyscalculia specifically and not on a broader population of low-achieving math students who may or may not have dyscalculia. Neuroscientific research that examines where processing is taking place in the brains of individuals with dyscalculia would support deeper understanding of this learning difference and could provide a starting point for a neurological basis for identifying strengths of dyscalculia. Much of the current research on dyscalculia is focused on students. More research is needed on the experience of dyscalculia in adulthood as well as in twice-exceptional populations. Additionally, research into effective educational interventions to support learning for those with dyscalculia is needed, including ways to incorporate practical, life skill–oriented strategies to support these individuals into adulthood. Finally, research is sorely needed that reframes the conversation so that the brains of those with dyscalculia can be viewed as different, rather than defective.

What Can YOU Do? Call to Action

It can feel overwhelming to know what to do or how to proceed, especially when faced with trying to navigate an educational system, and the world, with the challenges of a little-known and often poorly understood learning difference. Following is a breakdown of simple steps you can take to begin to effect change, with a nod to the popular metaphor, "Even a small ripple can become a great wave."

Educate Yourself

By educating yourself, you put yourself in a better position to be able to increase your own empathy, address your own misconceptions and those of others, and ultimately help to reduce harm. Suggested resources, including websites, books, and leading researchers, can be found in the resources list in Chapter 6.

Reduce Stigma Through Openness and Honesty

There tends to be a strong stigma surrounding learning differences, and depending on your cultural background, it can be exceedingly difficult to be open and honest about such differences, especially when they are viewed through a strong deficit lens. So what can you do to combat the stigma?

- As much as possible, reframe learning differences as a reflection of the natural diversity of humans, rather than a deficiency to be ashamed of or embarrassed by.
- Be a strong model for openness and acceptance, and foster safe and inclusive environments.
- Share your personal stories, or reference stories you've heard or read here, which can be a powerful tool for shifting perspectives.
- While context, relationships, comfort, and psychological safety will play a role in decisions about whether or not to disclose a learning difference, being open when it feels safe to do so can serve to foster self-acceptance,

strengthen relationships, and open the door for opportunities for individualized support and a more inclusive environment, while silence risks increased isolation, misunderstanding, shame, anxiety, and frustration.

Advocacy and Awareness

Advocacy is crucial for empowering individuals and groups, allowing their voices and experiences to be heard and respected, protecting rights and promoting equity, and influencing decision making that directly affects their lives. In his book, Brian Butterworth (2019) calls for systemic change, including improved awareness for the public and for those with the power to change policy. He supports efforts toward earlier identification, support and funding for further research, and changes to teacher training programs to better equip educators to support dyscalculic students.

Some practical steps you can take to be a strong advocate include:

- Speak up when necessary in all spaces where it is needed: schools, workplaces, and public spaces.
- Insist on comprehensive, research-based training and professional development for educators and other professionals who work with 2e/dyscalculic individuals that includes and prioritizes twice-exceptionality, dyscalculia, and inclusive curriculum design.
- Educate others. Butterworth (2019) cites lack of recognition as a factor in the slow pace of positive change. Share what you know, what you're learning, what your questions are. Share resources. Spread the word!

Embrace Neurodiversity in All Its Forms

Neurodiversity is a natural part of human variation and should be appreciated and valued. Simple actions you can take to spread understanding, appreciation, and acceptance include:

- Help others understand that differences in how people think, learn, process, and communicate are not

disorders—though they can certainly result in significant challenges in a neurotypical world.
- Frame dyscalculia in the context of the wider neurodiversity movement and include intersections with dyslexia, attention deficit hyperactivity disorder (ADHD), autism, and other learning differences.
- Challenge the deficit model, and help others to see the value in highlighting what's right, rather than what's wrong.
- Advocate for environments that are more inclusive for a wide range of people, and point to the value of cognitive diversity at home, school, the workplace, and communities in supporting a culture of innovation, compassion, and empathy.

Lead With Empathy

Real change starts with empathy. The experiences and stories shared by the study participants point not only to their misunderstood challenges and often over-looked strengths but also to the mental and emotional load of navigating a neurotypical world that wasn't created with their needs in mind and the resilience that helped them to pave their way through. When we lead with empathy, we approach others with curiosity rather than judgment, we listen without trying to fix, and we hold space for the experiences of others, even when they are vastly different from our own. Leading with empathy creates possibilities for deeper understanding, effective support, and stronger relationships grounded in dignity and respect.

Conclusion

This chapter began with challenges and limitations of the study and shifted to a forward-thinking call to action. While acknowledging areas for further investigation, particularly in the underexplored experiences of gifted adults with dyscalculia, the recommendations offered here shine a spotlight on the need for systemic change, wider awareness, and more inclusive practices and attitudes. Informed by participant voices and supported by current literature, the message is clear: it is time to shift the conversation from deficit to difference, from silence to advocacy, and from awareness to action. Small, intentional efforts—in classrooms, communities, or conversations—have the potential to create a lasting wave of change.

Closing Remarks

Research into the understanding of dyscalculia is growing but continues to fall short in comparison to what is known about other learning differences. In addition, in spite of studies showing the benefits of a strength-based view of learning differences, the research continues to view dyscalculia through a deficit lens. This multiple case study analysis was seeking to explore the experiences of gifted adults with dyscalculia and to begin to identify and shine a spotlight on their academic, cognitive, socioemotional, and creative strengths. The rich, personal stories shared by the participants ground these findings in real-world experience, providing a window into how gifted adults with dyscalculia navigate challenges while drawing on unique strengths. Deep gratitude is owed to these individuals for generously sharing their stories, which not only deepen our understanding but also humanize and add urgency to the call for a shift toward a strength-based understanding of dyscalculia as a cognitive difference with its own set of unique strengths.

References

Butterworth, B. (2019). *Can fish count? What animals reveal about our uniquely mathematical minds*. Basic Books.

Johnson, R. B. (2008). Interpretive validity. In L. M. Given (Ed.), *The Sage encyclopedia of qualitative research methods* (pp. 282–285). Sage Publications. https://doi.org/10.4135/9781412963909

About the Author

Ashleigh D'Aunoy, Ed.D., is a teacher and educational consultant specializing in gifted and twice-exceptional learners, with over 25 years of experience working with students from elementary school to the graduate level. She earned her doctorate in cognitive diversity in education from Bridges Graduate School, where her research focused on dyscalculia in gifted adults. As an educator, she is dedicated to building inclusive, strength-based programs for neurodiverse students. Outside of her professional work, she enjoys sharing good meals with friends, playing the flute, reading fiction, watching classic films, traveling, treasure-hunting in thrift stores, and spending time with her husband, Paul Conover, their adult son, Julien, and her rescue pug, Linus.

For Product Safety Concerns and Information please contact our EU representative GPSR@taylorandfrancis.com
Taylor & Francis Verlag GmbH, Kaufingerstraße 24, 80331 München, Germany

www.ingramcontent.com/pod-product-compliance
Lightning Source LLC
Chambersburg PA
CBHW070551170426
43201CB00012B/1805